Practical
Social Media for Dentists
And 50 Ideas for *Your* Practice

John Syrbu DDS

DEDICATION

To my best friend, Natalie.

CONTENTS

FOREWORD

There are three things I loved about John Syrbu's new book, *Practical Social Media for Dentists*.

First, John does an excellent job providing a brief historical background on advertising and the advent of social media that gives context to social media marketing in a dental practice. This will be especially helpful for practices just getting started because social media marketing requires a very different mindset than traditional advertising and marketing.

The second thing I really liked is John's observations about the characteristics of great content. Social media effectiveness inside a dental practice is largely dependent on creating content that people will find value in, and share. This is one of the biggest struggles for practices and John's explanation is spot-on relevant.

And third, his 50 specific ideas can easily become the foundation for a content calendar as team members map out their own practice's customized plan. Consistency is social media marketing's secret sauce and nearly every one of the ideas will help provide that consistency.

A great read!

Jack Hadley
Partner, *My Social Practice*

1 HOW WE GOT HERE

D o you ever wonder how you got here? You, a dentist, having to keep up with "social media". It seems silly. Depending on when you started practicing, you probably didn't see yourself updating your status with Facebook or tweeting on Twitter. But whether you like it or not, social media has become commonplace and a key piece of the modern day marketing puzzle. It has become an integral part of our daily communication. And in order to better understand our current situation, it may be helpful to consider the major events and developments that led us to this point.

For a large portion of history, print was the only medium available. The invention of the moveable type, or Gutenberg press, in 1450 made mass printing possible. In the 1700's, magazines emerged, later to become a vector for niche marketing. The 19th century saw its first paid advertisement run in the French newspaper *La Presse* in 1836, allowing the paper to lower its price, expand its distribution and increase profitability. It didn't take long for every major news source to adopt this formula. Posters also became so popular that they were banned on private property in London in 1839. Decades later, the earliest recorded billboard rentals popped up in towns and along major roadways in 1867. Visual advertising through each medium captured the eyes of their consumers.

Starting in 1922, radio advertising appealed to another sensory modality of the public – their ears. Families gathered nightly in their living rooms to listen to the radio, which made its way into over half of American households by 1933.

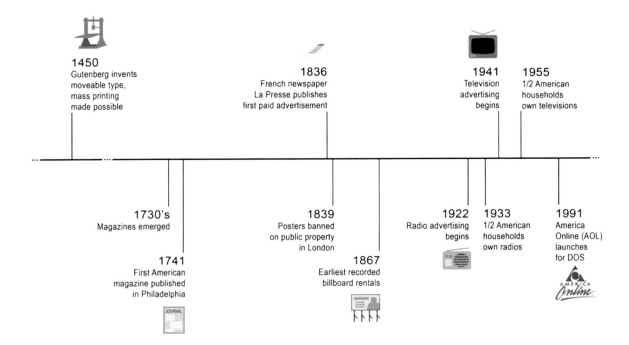

1450
Gutenberg invents moveable type, mass printing made possible

1836
French newspaper La Presse publishes first paid advertisement

1941
Television advertising begins

1955
1/2 American households own televisions

1730's
Magazines emerged

1839
Posters banned on public property in London

1922
Radio advertising begins

1933
1/2 American households own radios

1991
America Online (AOL) launches for DOS

1741
First American magazine published in Philadelphia

1867
Earliest recorded billboard rentals

In 1941, marketers infiltrated television sets, which combined auditory and visual appeal for their consumers. As radio ad revenue slowly but steadily declined by approximately 2% annually, a sharper decline of 9% was noted in 1954. In the same year, TV ad revenue grew from 5% to 15% to surpass both radio and magazine ad revenue. By 1955, over half of U.S. households owned a television set. Over the next few decades, televisions continued to grow in popularity and prominence, eventually displacing even newspapers as the nation's largest ad medium.

Several decades later, the marketing world once again grew a new branch with the introduction of personal computers and the rise of the internet.

The early 1990's fostered internet and e-mail advertising techniques, a time when you excitedly and eagerly awaited the phrase *"You've got mail!"* Meanwhile, new technologies continued to emerge and become adopted by wide audiences, such as mobile phones.

The latter half of the 90's also gave rise to search engines such as Yahoo and Google, which helped users find the information, products and services they desired. At their inception, search algorithms relied on webmaster-provided information such as meta data, keyword density and other on-page factors. Google later introduced PageRank, the metric used to determine a website's rank within a search, to include a function of the quality and strength of inbound links from outside sources as well as on-page factors. Therein the term *search engine optimization*, or SEO, was born.

As internet marketing continued to grow and the dot-com bubble burst on March 10, 2000, consumers gained traction and began to push back against disruptive outbound marketing tactics. For example, in 2003, the CAN-SPAM act was signed into law, setting national standards against sending unsolicited commercial e-mails. Personalized search results on Google were informed by a user's past search history. The internet persistently and progressively shifted the tides toward inbound marketing characterized by an emphasis on information sharing and user-centered function, design and collaboration.

If you are unfamiliar with outbound versus inbound marketing techniques, let's take a moment to consider the differences. In general, *outbound marketing* is considered the old-fashioned, more traditional mode of business whereby a company pushes products or services down a one-way street unto the customer. Businesses will pursue or solicit customers through print, radio, banner and TV ads or even cold calls (think Yellow Pages, billboards and direct mailing). *Inbound marketing*, on the other hand, caters to the needs and preferences of the consumer. Essentially, businesses earn people's interest rather than purchase it. Communication is an interactive two-

way street. With inbound marketing, customers often seek businesses via search engines, referrals and social media. Inbound marketing often aims to entertain and educate customers, providing value rather than direct advertisement. Inbound marketing techniques also cost approximately 62% less when compared with outbound marketing, with about a 60% decrease in cost per lead with inbound marketing.[1]

Outbound Marketing	Inbound Marketing
• Communication is a one-way street	• Interactive, two-way communication
• Businessess seek customers via print, TV, radio, banner advertisements, and cold calls	• Costomers find businesses via search engines, referrals, social media and personal research
• Businesses distribute advertisements	• Businesses seek to educate, entertain and provide value to customer
• Rarely provide value	

Now, which modality sounds more like dentistry? From an internal marketing standpoint, I am of the opinion that the dental profession has been practicing inbound marketing for decades. We present our findings to our patients, educate them of the risks and benefits of various treatment options and together we determine which treatment option is the right one for them. More on this later.

---

[1] *2012 Report on Inbound marketing practices & trends.* Hubspot, 2012.

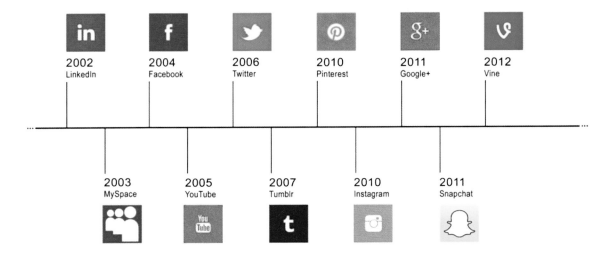

2002 LinkedIn | 2004 Facebook | 2006 Twitter | 2010 Pinterest | 2011 Google+ | 2012 Vine

2003 MySpace | 2005 YouTube | 2007 Tumblr | 2010 Instagram | 2011 Snapchat

Enter LinkedIn (2002), MySpace (2003) and Facebook (2004), websites that provided customized profiles and platforms to network personally and/or professionally with other users online. Based on membership and popularity, Facebook pulled ahead to become the most prominent of the social media sites, and usership today exceeds 1.4 billion worldwide. While it may be impressive that more than 1 out of 7 people in the world use Facebook, the numbers are even more relevant locally, where 74% of online adults are also using social media as of January 2014.[1] Heck, 48% of 18-34 year olds check Facebook when they wake up, with 28% doing so before even getting out of bed![2]

With such remarkable growth and popularity, other social media platforms

began to surface – Twitter (2006), Pinterest (2010), Instagram (2010), Snapchat (2011), etc. One by one they emerged, each bringing a slightly different twist on social interactions, and each accumulating hundreds of millions of active users. Still, Facebook reigns king in terms of total users and monthly active users (MAU's). If the internet put the keys in the ignition for inbound marketing, social media put the pedal to the metal, allowing customers to interact with businesses in new and exciting ways.

Meanwhile, two important trends were taking form. The first was the incredible growth and availability of cellular phones. By 2010, 90% of U.S. households had a cell phone. The year after, 1 in 2 Americans owned a smartphone, and time spent on the internet surpassed time spent watching television. In fact, many consumers today are participating in the *second-*

---

[1] Pew Research Center, January 2014.

[2] Facebook Statistics, Stats and Facts for 2011. www.digitalbuzzblog.com.

screen phenomenon, where a mobile device, such as a smartphone or tablet, is used to provide an enhanced or interactive experience during linear content such as television programming. Some call it "social television". By now you've seen shows that feature live conversations with their audiences via Twitter, or feature hashtags (#'s) for textual and visual commentary. It can even be argued that the smartphone or tablet has actually evolved to be our "first" screen, leaving the television and desktop behind. Social media has latched onto and altered or enhanced practically every other media platform, from print to radio and television.

The second trend is that other forms of digital marketing were losing their luster. By 2010, banner advertisement click-through rates had dropped to 0.1% according to Google, down from 0.5% in the early 2000's and 3.0% in the mid-1990's[3]. In 2011, e-mail open rates were at about 17%, down from 26% in 2009 and 37.3% in 2002.[4,5] Which should come as no surprise given that 90% of emails in 2010 were reported as "spam". In fact Google's e-mail service, G-Mail, now automatically separates your inboxes into *Primary, Social* and *Promotions* folders. You don't even see the *Social* and *Promotions* e-mails unless you specifically open those folders or individually designate e-mail from any sender in the *Social* or *Promotions* folder to appear in the *Primary* inbox. Another display of consumer-centered design and function, in effect a repellant for spam and interruptive marketing – a recurring theme that plays throughout this text.

While a plethora of social media services exist today, Facebook remains by far the largest, most prominent and most relevant social media platform for small businesses. In June of 2012, about 8 million businesses had created Facebook pages. That number doubled by May of 2013 and upwards of 30 million businesses ran Facebook pages as of June 2014. As such most of the social media content and advice in this book is set within the context of your Facebook presence. However, social is social. The underlying message and themes of quality content will be successful across various platforms. In fact, many of the social media platforms, such as Twitter and LinkedIn, have slowly migrated to a more Facebook-esc appearance and user experience, allowing pictures and video on a scrollable wall or news feed of some sort. This trend is affectionately termed *Facebookification*.

Still, we outline the key and sometimes subtle differences of all currently relevant social media platforms in Chapter 8 of this book. After all, "If content is king, then context is God". In order for your content to exert maximum

---

[3] *Thorson & Schumann*. October 2004.

[4] *Harte-Hanks*. June 2011.

[5] *DoubleClick by Google*. Q3 2002.

impact, it must be optimized and tailored to the unique characteristics and features of the given social media outlet.

Social media is here to stay. It has integrated seamlessly into various aspects of our everyday lives and ignoring it is no longer an option. Now that we have a better idea of basic marketing principles and how social media come to be, let's take a look at the role it plays for our practice and how we can incorporate it into our playbook.

"Social media is here to stay."

2 THE ROLE OF FACEBOOK

Some marketers will attest that a business's social media outlets are more influential than their website. Especially for small businesses. And your practice, no matter how big or small, or even if you own several, is a small business. I won't arm wrestle you for it, but I will say that these days, your website and social media go hand in hand. It's your horse and your carriage, your bread and your butter. And for optimal results, you'll want to maximize your potential with both.

Author Simon Sinek gave a popular TED Talk and wrote a book on the concept of *the golden circle.*[6] If you haven't at least watched the presentation, pull it up on YouTube when you have a minute. Sinek argues that modern successful ideas share a pattern that is rooted in human decision-making. He stated that great leaders inspire action by starting with and placing an emphasis on their "why". That's their passion or motivation, what gets them up in the morning and the reason they do what they do. Then they present their "how". This is the process, steps or methods involved. And finally, the product or the "what" is unveiled.

---

[6] *Start With Why: How Great Leaders Inspire Everyone to Take Action*. Simon Sinek, 2009.

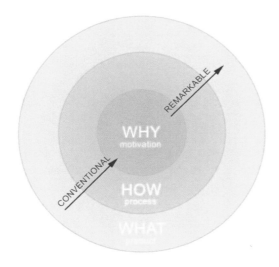

More and more, brands and businesses are touting their "why" and their "how" above their "what". By that I mean people, consumers and patients alike, care an awful lot about why you're doing something and how you go about it. Transparency is a growing component in the decision making process of today's consumers. Let's consider some simple examples. Ten years ago, the words "organic" and "free-range" or "grass-fed" weren't stamped all over the expensive cartons of eggs. Cosmetics companies that don't utilize animal testing are seen as caring companies whose humane practices say as much about them as their makeup. Apple has built an entire empire and a cultural following based on its passion for design and function. All of these products tend to cost more than their conventional counterparts, but that hasn't stopped consumers from flocking to them.

In terms of dental marketing, your website is your "what". A relatively stagnant entity, it provides the most basic and objective information about the office, i.e. your name, your address, business hours and hopefully brief profiles of your staff along with a few pictures of the office. All perfectly staged and polished, as they should be.

"But I have a regularly updated blog on my website" you might say, "with this, patients know that I am passionate about my work". And that's good. But while that boosts your SEO rankings, none of your patients are curling up by the fireplace to read about your periodontal services. Even if you personally hand-write each article, prospective patients won't gain insight to your personality, your day-to-day interactions or the atmosphere of your office. And these days, *that's* important.

Your social media outlets are your "why". With an emphasis on transparency, education and entertainment, they provide a glimpse into the true colors of your practice. Social media is a public display of your values and community, and provides another avenue of discovery and communication for new, old and prospective patients alike. Sound familiar? That's inbound marketing.*

---

*If "inbound marketing" is a new term at this point, head back over to Chapter 1 – no skipping ahead!

MEET KAREN

To illustrate this point, let's consider a scenario between Karen and three dentists, Drs. A, B and C. Karen is currently a *prospective* patient. She recently moved to Sampletown, USA where her husband works for the city and she got a position with Generic-Co. Karen's husband is 40 years old while Karen is a millennial in her 30's with two children. As an aside, they happen to have dual-coverage dental insurance.

In the past few weeks she has received fliers from several dentists in town. One of them may have been from Dr. A or Dr. B, but she didn't commit any to memory as she was still settling into her new home. Being a millennial, Karen is accustomed to doing her own research for most products and services, so she opens her browser and Googles "Sampletown Dentist".

Ⓐ **Dr. A Dental**
www.drAdental.com
4.7 ★★★★✦ 12 Google reviews · Google+ page

Ⓑ **Dr. B, DDS**
www.drBdds.com
4.8 ★★★★★ 6 Google reviews · Google+ page

Ⓒ **Dr. C Family Dentistry**
www.drCfamilydentistry.com
4.7 ★★★★✦ 12 Google reviews · Google+ page

Dr. A is first on the list, Dr. B is second and Dr. C is third. Karen opened all three websites on separate tabs within her browser. She gave them each a once-over and within less than a minute she had it narrowed down to Drs. A and C. She tried to click a link in Dr. B's website, who was second on Google, but the website was outdated and the link was defective. Two strikes and he's out. Just like that. Wait, does it really happen like that? You bet.

Karen wants at least two dentists to chose from, so let's compare Drs. A and C. They both have good websites. In fact they both have *great* websites. They're easy on the eyes with a pleasant color palate. The Docs present themselves professionally with a hint of personality and brand identity splashed in. Each website is finely polished with professional photos of the doctors and staff, and no spelling or grammatical errors appear anywhere on either site. Both doctors seem to have good reputations, as both showcase reviews and testimonials from patients on their sites.

By now a habit, Karen clicks the familiar blue "f" at the bottom of Dr. A's site to check out their Facebook page. It lacks luster. The profile photo is an image of the practice's roadway sign in their front lawn, and the cover photo is a pixelated image of the office building. As Karen scrolls through some recent posts, the identity of the practice is lost on her. The posts are inconsistent. A cartoon here and there, pictures without captions and a few written status updates soliciting patients to call or schedule appointments. Hardly any faces to be seen and the dates on the posts were also sparse – weeks, sometimes months apart. Little was gained from this experience, leaving Karen feeling a bit empty.

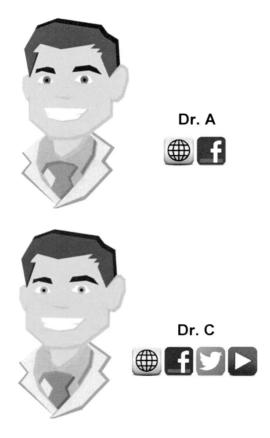

Dr. A

Dr. C

Dr. C's Facebook page, whose link is found at the top of his website, offered some contrast. Dr. C features his office building with a clear blue sky as his profile picture and a professional group photo of the staff as a cover photo. Crisp, colorful images fill the page. The posts date several days apart, the most recent post from yesterday showed a smiling hygienist holding what looked like a birthday cupcake with Dr. C.

Other photos feature various staff members with patients, some of them children with "perfect check-ups" and gift giveaways. Some humorous posts, holiday posts and even a few educational posts with dental tips are easily spotted with a few scrolls of Karen's finger. In just a minute or two, Karen was able to appreciate the atmosphere and personality of the dental office. She felt like she knew the staff, or would at least be able to recognize some of them, without ever having met them. Social media gave Karen another dimension and avenue to compare her options. And it solidified her decision to call Dr. C's office.

And that's if Karen didn't have an established social network of friends in town. I've seen several of my personal friends simply post a question to their friends saying "I need a new dentist. Anyone have any recommendations?" The suggestions from their friends and the reasons for their recommendations were very insightful. Many of them involved the personality, atmosphere and environment of the named offices, dentists and/or staff. Interestingly, none of them cited the qualifications of their dentists or the margins of their restorations.

After coming in for an appointment, Karen has upgraded from a prospective patient to a *new* patient. Since she enjoyed her experience with you and your staff, she went on to "like" your page on Facebook. She saw a sign in the reception area prompting her to do so and informing patients of the benefits of staying updated with your social media account(s). The social icons were on your business card as well as the *Welcome* or *Thank You* card you sent to Karen's family after their first visit. A staff member may also have casually mentioned it in conversation at some point.

Your steady stream of personable and pleasant content has made Karen feel comfortable with you and your staff in record time. Karen is now a *current* patient. Social media keeps you and Karen connected. If someone asks about her dentist, she can vouch for your office. With Karen's recommendation, you have gone from top-of-mind to tip-of-tongue.

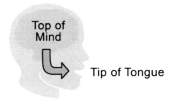

THE POWER OF SOCIAL

We know that word of mouth is the most powerful and effective form of marketing. I've got good news for you – social media marketing *is* word of mouth marketing. Its potential is particularly potent on social media for two reasons. First and foremost is that the message comes from your friends or family.

Whether or not they have an informed decision, it has a certain influence on you. Second is that if a patient mentions you or engages with your content, a variable number of *their* friends may see the interaction on their news feed. So rather than the "one-on-one" interaction of word of mouth, social media can become a "one-to-many" interaction.

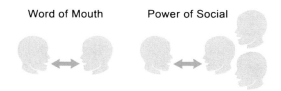

The average user on Facebook has a personal network of about 300 friends. Even if you get as few as 300 of your patients to like you on Facebook (your goal should be *much* higher) and each one of them has 300 friends – you have a potential market of 90,000 people who you can promote a word of mouth referral to. It's easy to visualize the potential for social media's role within your external marketing strategy. It's even easier to understand its role in internal marketing.

ACROSS GENERATIONS

Social media is a standard form of communication within the millennial generation, and growing in influence among Generation X and Baby Boomers alike. Let's consider these broad cohorts, their differences and their similarities.

Millennials were born between 1980-2000 and age between 15-35 years old. They have grown up during a time of rapid change and are considered the first "digitally native" generation. They also represent the largest of the groups, a whopping 92 million strong in the United States.[7] While they are devoted to health, wellness and the environment, you will have to work hardest for their business as they turn to brands that offer maximum convenience at the lowest cost. And with lower employment levels and ever increasing debt, they may have less money to spend.[8,9] But millennials not only shape today's market trends, they also represent the future of the dental industry.

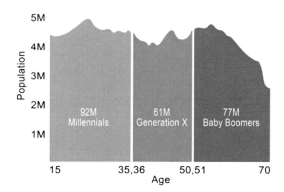

Generation X'ers are aged 36-50 and the Baby Boomers are 51-70 years in age. They represent about 61 million and 77 million of the U.S. population, respectively. Orthodontists and pediatric dentists aside, they also represent the majority of your patients. Want to know how to market to Generation X and Baby Boomers? Learn to market to millennials and you're covered. Why? Because modern day society is obsessed with looking, feeling and acting younger. 40 is the new 30. 50 is the new 40, and so forth. Don't get me wrong, of course a large portion of your dentistry is being performed on the elder two generations. But in terms of effective marketing tactics, you'll want to master the mediums that are being utilized and popularized by the millennial generation.

Even orthodontists and pediatric dentists should be marketing to millennials, given their target audience of young mothers. Recall that at its inception, the original users of Facebook in 2004 and 2005 were college students. While teenagers in the 13-20 year old age group turn to other storytelling apps like Instagram and Snapchat, Facebook's early adopters and loyal user base are maturing to perfectly coordinate with the target audience, the parents of these children and teenagers.

And if your practice is primarily comprised of the Baby Boomer generation, get this – Facebook's fastest growing user cohort was recently shown to be – ages 65 and up.[10]

[7] US Census Bureau

[8] Bureau of Labor Statistics

[9] Federal Reserve

[10] Pew Research Center Internet Project, 2013.

Ideally as a general dentist, you have a broad and healthy mix of patients. Even if you think you can retire with your aging patient population, you may be limiting your office's potential. When you move to sell your practice, a young dentist may not be eager to treat solely elder patients that think he or she is too young to know what they are doing. And the value of the practice will drop accordingly.

THE SERVICE INDUSTRY

You purchased your phone or your car to obtain a product, i.e. the phone, the car. You purchased it based on its features, recommendations, the price and so forth. And you probably don't know any of the people that made those products. In part because machines manufactured may of the parts and pieces, but also because Apple or Honda are in the business of making products. Dentistry, on the other hand, is a service industry. The friendly and familiar faces of the dental team provide the service of dentistry. And the key to any service business is *relationships*.

Many practices exert vast amounts of time and energy on acquiring new patients. If their chairs aren't full to the brim they'll open the front door and lose focus of their existing patients, often leaving the back door wide open. While social media can play an important role in capturing the interest of new patients, it plays an equally important role in your internal marketing strategy as a means for patient retention. After all, followers of your social media outlets will consist almost exclusively of current patients of the practice.

Think of the patient whose main interaction with your office is a cleaning every six or twelve months and the occasional minor restorative work. What's keeping them from getting a coupon in the mail for a cheaper cleaning at another dentist's office? Ideally, the internal marketing that you've achieved with the atmosphere of the office, the interaction with your staff, etc. would be enough. However, six to twelve months is a long time. Think of your classmates or old friends that you only see once or twice a year. If it weren't for Facebook and other social media platforms, how often would those friends come to mind? Not very often, and that's a *friend*. Consistent engagement on social media helps to cement the relationship between your office and your patient. Having a patient like or follow your page enhances your identity as *their* dentist.

As we've seen with the evolution of marketing media, today's society values transparency. Social media has helped to personify businesses and open the door for more effective and efficient communication between brands and consumers, doctors and patients, etc. Social media answers the ever important question of "why" and can help strengthen the relationship between new, current and especially prospective patients. Our sample patient, Karen, was a millennial. While our patients may represent all three generations discussed, our marketing efforts should align with the ideals of inbound marketing principles that have proven to be effective with the millennial generation. Next, let's take a look at best practices when constructing your Facebook page and building your online empire.

"Social media is your why."

3 THE SETUP

W hether you're creating your practice's Facebook page for the very first time or looking to improve your current page, this chapter will help you develop your Facebook following. I encourage even seasoned social media veterans to read through this chapter to obtain tips on various aspects of creating and maintaining stronger relationships with your patients. I will be brief on the more self-explanatory elements and elaborate where special attention and consideration is warranted.

CREATING A FACEBOOK PAGE

1. Sign into your Facebook account and go to Pages → Create A Page or go to www.facebook.com/pages/create.

2. Click "Local Business or Page".

3. Fill in the required information.
   a. Most dentists choose the category of "Doctor".
   b. Your Business or Place Name is simply the name of the practice. Do not include any subtitles, slogans or descriptors here.
   c. Continue with your Street Address, City/State, Zip Code and Phone.
   d. Agree to Facebook's Page Terms.

4. The About section is fairly straight forward.
   a. Under Category you may enter "Dentist".
   b. Your Description is a short summary statement for your practice. You will have the chance

to input a longer description later in the process. Keep this one short and sweet.

c. Enter your website URL.

d. Choose "Yes" for the remaining questions as your dental practice is a real establishment and you are authorized to represent yourself on Facebook.

5. Common and appropriate profile pictures for a dental practice include, but are not limited to:
   - your practice name and logo
   - a photo of the doctor(s)
   - the entire dental staff
   - your building
   - the reception area if it is particularly inviting, etc.

Whatever you chose for your profile picture, make sure it is a high-quality image. Pictures taken by a professional photographer work well. I do *not* recommended using stock photos, pictures of patients, treatment rooms (no matter how cool you might think yours are), dental equipment or photos with text in the image. You want an image that is quick and easy to view, as it will mostly appear as a small thumbnail on your patient's News Feed. Viewers associate your profile picture with your practice, so make it simple and pleasant.

Keep in mind that your profile picture is not a stagnant entity. For example, refresh the theme or colors in your profile picture with the seasons and/or in the weeks before your favorite holidays. We do this with our personal profiles, don't leave your practice out of the fun.

6. Click "Add to Favorites". This will place your page on the left side of your screen for easy access anytime you sign into Facebook.

7. Next Facebook will ask you to create an ad to get more people to like your newly created Page. Facebook advertising can be a reasonably priced option to bring awareness to your social media presence. Facebook advertisements allow you to effectively reach your target audience by providing options to filter hits to any city in the United States. Facebook also allows you to target ads by age, gender and even by people's interests listed on Facebook. However, it is way too early to think about Facebook advertisements. For now, click to skip.

8. Once you've opted out of advertising, you've completed the most basic setup, but we're not quite done yet. There are still a number of key elements that need to be addressed before you're ready for your debut.

Facebook will prompt you to "like" your own page, which you should do. Even if you aren't the one running the daily activities of the page, you'll be checking in from time to time. In addition, several administrators can be assigned to any Facebook page, while only the creator of the page can edit a page's settings.

9. Go to either "Admin Panel" → Edit Page → Update Page Info or scroll down to your page front to find "Update Page Info".

Here you will find a number of important features. The features listed in gray appear this way because you have likely already filled them out during the initial page setup.

a. Name

b. Facebook Wed Address: This is a custom web address for your page that Facebook provides free of charge. Essentially it is a Facebook-specific domain name that you can claim in the form of www.facebook.com/YourPractice. You are free to choose any address as long as it has not already been taken. Try to keep it short and intuitive. Most dentists either choose to name it after their practice, e.g. www.facebook.com/ClintonSmiles or by location and keyword, e.g. www.facebook.com/ClintonDentist. Facebook may require you to confirm your mobile phone number at this step.

c. Category

d. Subcategory

e. Address

f. Start Info

g. Hours: Enter your office hours. Make sure they are accurate and stay *updated*. Especially if you are a newer practice or have made any changes to your office hours recently. Facebook currently allows for weekly hours, so if you are open every other Saturday, you may need to include that in your description.

h. Short Description

i. Long Description: Feel free to elaborate on your practice, your mission statement or even give an overview for the types of treatments you provide here. But stay on topic, and keep it to two-three paragraphs. While most people won't read this section, even those that do will skip it if it's too lengthy.

j. Price Range: This pertains to restaurants mostly. Leave this section blank. You don't want to scare anyone away with your prices!

k. Parking: You may choose from street, parking lot or valet parking options. You do not need to fill this section out either, however if your practice does offer valet parking, then by all means let us know!

l. Phone

m. Email: Your practice should have an email address. If it doesn't – get one.

n. Website: List your website URL.

o. Official Page: This section does not pertain to most dentists, but simply states that if you are not the official spokesperson for your organization, you may declare the official representation here. This may come into play if individual dentists or other personnel have their own Facebook page(s) and would like to tie those pages to the practice's page.

10. You're almost there! The last step in your setup is your cover photo. Your cover photo is the backdrop to your page front and should be considered just as important as your profile picture. Like your profile picture, your cover photo may include your practice name and logo, a photo of the dentists and staff, the building or reception area. Your cover photo should *not* be the same image as your profile picture. Avoid placing small or excessive text in your cover photo as well. Think of this display as a store front or a book cover. Text may not even be legible on a standard smartphone screen. It should be visually captivating, not a chore to look

through. And do not attempt to put the names of the dentists, the address of the practice or the phone number in these images. It's tacky. Besides, if your patients want your number, they'll have no problem finding it.

Also keep in mind that your cover photo is rectangular (dimensions below) and your profile picture will overlap slightly at the bottom left corner, so keep the important components of your cover photo towards the right of the photo.

PROFILE AND COVER PHOTO DIMENSIONS

For the Photoshop experts in the room, below are the dimensions and specifications of the profile and cover photos. If your dimensions are off, Facebook will simply crop the photo and let you reposition the image to fill the space.

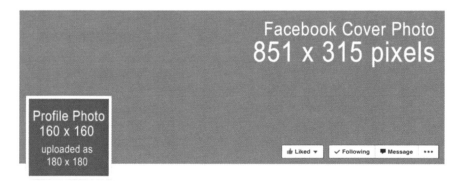

CALL TO ACTION BUTTON

In December, 2014 Facebook rolled out a "Call-To-Action" button for business pages. Intended to bring a business's main objective to the forefront of its Facebook page, the Call-To-Action button provides fans a quick link to the destination of your choice. The options are as follows:

- Book Now
- Contact Us
- Use App
- Play Game
- Shop Now
- Sign Up
- Watch Video

For most practices, the "Book Now" and "Contact Us" options are the most logical actions. However, if your practice has an app for your patients, you may direct them to the app. Or if you recorded a new promotional or educational video, you may want to market the video for some time thereafter with "Watch Video".

BUILD IT BEFORE THEY COME

Remember the phrase, "If you build it, they will come"? That doesn't really apply here, or hardly anywhere anymore. Perhaps if you're the only dentist in a high-need area. But where people have options, you'll need to do some marketing. And like your teeth, you'll want to have a solid foundation before you start building the house. The principles here can be applied to a new Facebook page as well as one that is being revitalized from a dormant state. First let's consider who will be creating and/or posting content to the page.

PAGE ADMINISTRATORS

Often times dentists appoint all Facebook responsibilities to a younger assistant, hygienist or other office member. This sounds like a good idea for two mains reasons. First, many dentists either don't feel comfortable using social media or they are not willing to put in the time and effort required to master the art. This is understandable given the workload required to run a productive dental practice. Second, many dentists assume that their younger employees simply "get it" and will know what to do. Not always the case.

Marketing is a field of study all on its own, of which social media is a relatively new branch. Like dentistry, it is an art and a science. Most of these entrusted employees' only experience with social media is having a personal Facebook account of their own. The question then becomes: do they have what it takes to effectively build your brand, represent the practice online and create, find and share engaging content that offers value to patients on a consistent basis?

A great place to start is to have *all*

page administrators read this text, including the doctor(s) in the practice. As the dentist, you need to be involved with your social media presence regardless of whether or not you are the one posting to the page. At a minimum, you need to check in with the page on a weekly (ideally daily) basis to review posted content as well as engagement received from your patients, i.e. likes, comments, shares, tags, reviews, check-ins and messages to the page. You don't want a patient compliment to go unnoticed. Or one to inquire when they might hear back from the message they sent last week. Your deer-in-headlights look will shine through anything you might be able to muster up on the spot. Alternatively you don't want to let any content linger that you disagree with or that does not represent the practice well. Neglect can also harm your ratings. Keep in mind that social media is a public platform. If a written complaint goes unaddressed, you are not doing your part in reputation management. Social media is a collaborative effort and a culture that should be created and cultivated within the office.

Let's say you do have someone in the office with a contagious personality who is digitally savvy and even has some experience in retail marketing. She's constantly taking pictures of everyone and everything around her, including herself! We'll call her Susie. You decide that Susie would be right for the job and designate her as a page administrator, in charge of running your

practice's Facebook page. If Susie is to be successful, she'll put in the hours and develop meaningful relationships to attract new patients and strengthen loyalty with her personable interactions. Hopefully Susie runs off of steam and pats on the back, because Susie will quickly find out that creating and maintaining a successful social media presence is a job that can be, well, a job!

My point is that maintaining a successful and engaging Facebook page is time-consuming, especially with an active group of hundreds, or better yet thousands, of Facebook fans. If Susie is your assistant and stays busy throughout the day with your patients and procedures, Susie is now working overtime for the practice. Some financial incentive or show of appreciation for a job well done is appropriate and strongly recommended (I've got your back, Susie!).

For this and other reasons, some dental practices have outsourced a portion of their social media responsibilities to hired professionals. There's nothing wrong with that as it's certainly not easy putting out quality, relevant content on a weekly basis. However, *NO* social media service should be providing *ALL* of your social media content and interaction. It is simply an impersonal feat that is doomed to fail. Remember that personality counts. The people, features and characteristics of your practice is unique to your practice. That's your identity and that's who your patients come to see, whether it's for their cleaning or for a break from their day while they're on Facebook. Feature your unique brand often. And a final word to the wise – content created specifically for dentists and generic content marketed towards dentists are two different things. Choose any co-managers of your social media account(s) with some discretion.

That being said, it is a scalable feat to manage your own social media presence internally. For some practices, the best way to tackle these responsibilities is to distribute them. In fact this is the most efficient way to go about it. Social media is a team sport. Facebook allows page creators to appoint various positions to their page administrators, and there's no limit to the number of administrators you can assign. Available roles currently include Admin, Editor, Moderator, Advertiser and Insight Analyst. Each of these roles have different access capabilities and privileges. Large corporations have full-time employees filling each of these positions, while your practice may have any combination of team member roles. The process is:

1. To add an administrator, find the *Settings* tab on the top right screen within the Admin Panel. Click on *Page Roles*.

2. Search for the new administrator from within your Facebook friends (you should be Facebook friends with your team) or type in their email address.

3. Choose a role for the new administrator from the drop-down menu.

The roles to choose from are as follows:

Admin: Can manage all aspects of the Page including sending messages and posting as the Page, creating ads, seeing which admin created a post or comment, viewing insights and assigning Page roles.

Editor: Can edit the Page, send messages and post as the Page, create ads, see which admin created a post or comment and view insights.

Moderator: Can respond to and delete comments on the Page, send messages as the Page, see which admin created a post or comment, create ads and view insights.

Advertiser: Can see which admin created a post or comment, create ads and view insights.

Analyst: Can see which admin created a post or comment and view insights.

Getting more people involved is a great way to maximize your engagement potential and alleviate some of the costs of staying active in your virtual network. If your staff dynamic permits for adding more administrators to the Facebook page, get as many people involved as your comfort level and their motivation allows. Use your judgment, and do not force anyone to get involved, as some personalities and character traits simply do not translate well on social media.

Susie, as we noted earlier, is perfect

for social media. Cathy, Stacy and Steve might also be interested in getting involved. If they're up for the job, have them read this book. Once everyone is on board with the basic rules and the message you want to convey, make them administrators and have some fun with it! Heard of "Employee of the Month"? In the corporate world, it symbolizes employee appreciation, boosts morale and can even lead to higher production. Host a "Most Engaging Staff" contest between your staff members with a fun new prize every month. Likes get 1 point, comments get 2 and shares are worth 5. The "Facebook Insights" feature will tell you exactly how much engagement each of your posts accomplished (see Chapter 7).

YOUR FIRST POSTS

You are now ready to create your first set of posts. "What? I don't even have any Facebook fans yet! Why would I waste my time?" You're right, you may not have any fans aside from your staff at this point, and maybe a few of their friends that trickled in when they saw them "like" your new page. However, your page may be completely empty at this point. You wouldn't invite all of your friends over for a cocktail party to an empty house with no food, furniture or decoration.

Or even if you've been present but static on Facebook for some time, you aren't quite ready to launch a campaign for your patients to follow your page.

Each of your posts have a date on them. If there hasn't been any recent activity or the posts are few and far between, that sends the wrong message. You may not think it's important, but people will see that and question the value in publicly "liking" your page.

So let's get a few posts on the wall. Start with a post today. Post again the day after tomorrow. Then again next week. What should you post? We'll spend the next few chapters discussing Facebook content. But these first few posts are just to get the ball rolling. While conversational posts or open-ended questions might be appropriate when you have a solid following, your first posts will be simple statements and tidbits. You don't have anyone to interact with or fans to share your content yet, so these will be freebies. They should be interesting, but no need to put out your best work.

You can start with staff photos and scenic shots of your office. You can even create albums for each titled "Our Team" or "Office Tour". Next find a comic, talk about a holiday or wish your local high school basketball team good luck at their regional game. Have staff "like" or "comment" on some of these posts, just to fill the space and break the silence. Once you have a healthy handful of posts, at least enough to fill the initial screen when you first open your page, you are ready for the next step.

FAMILY FIRST

Next let's invite your friends and family, as well as the friends and family of staff to like the page. "Oh come on! Isn't this for patients?" That's next. First we invite family and friends to build our foundation. Meanwhile Facebook posts should continue to be posted at a relatively consistent rate of 2-3 posts per week. Now that we have the food out, some furniture and decorations on the wall, we're letting the first few guests into the party. Assuming your family and friends like you, they might "like" some of your ongoing content. This is your social media presence in the budding stages.

It should also be noted that if you are making a coordinated effort to join several social media outlets, such as Twitter or Instagram, you can use a similar approach. But because these platforms operate differently, it may not be the same *exact* approach. Other social media platform considerations are discussed in Chapter 8.

YOUR SOCIAL DEBUT

Now that you are ready to make your debut, plan your campaign appropriately. This includes signs and other internal marketing tactics, one-on-one marketing or word-of-mouth and Facebook advertisements.

Although some patients will intuitively search for you on Facebook out of habit, many won't. The goal is to make it easy for them to do so. Have free Wi-fi waiting for them in the reception area and treatment rooms. If you insist on a password-protected network, have signs informing patients of the password in common areas. On the same poster or a nearby sign, inform patients of the social media platforms where you can be found. The association between "free Wi-fi" and social media does not have to be subtle.

Aside from simply saying "Like us on Facebook" or "Follow us on Twitter," market the benefits or perks of following your practice on Facebook or Twitter, such as contests and giveaways, monthly drawings for prizes, special offers or discounts and promotions, etc. Place one of these signs at the front desk where patients check in and check out. The benefit of this location is that every patient stops here and where your patients converse with your front desk staff. It's a visual and a great segue to mentioning the Facebook page. Other good locations include the chairs by your magazines, common hallways and even hygiene or treatment rooms. When you leave the room for an exam, patients sometimes look to your walls and posters to pass the time.

Advertising your social media presence should also be readily displayed on various printed materials and online outlets. Include the well-known social media logos of the platforms that you use on all signs, business cards, welcome and thank you cards, posters, etc. Make the social media buttons on your website quick and easy to find. Tie your social media presence to your brand's identity.

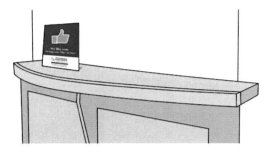

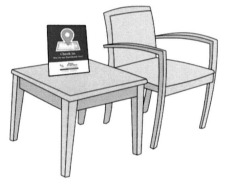

Some practices incorporate Facebook referrals into other realms of their internal marketing strategy. For example, a practice may use punch cards or other scoring methods to "gamify" their marketing efforts. The idea is that any patient can obtain a punch card from the office. They accumulate punches or points and trade them in for various prizes, from white strips and free cleanings to gift cards and electronics. A sample score card may look as follows:

★2   6-month check-up (each)
★1   Perfect check-up (no cavities)
★2   Facebook like, Twitter follow, etc.
★5   Write a Review
     (Yelp, Google, Facebook)
★20 Refer a friend/family
     (awarded at their scheduled appt)

As mentioned, word-of-mouth is one of the most powerful marketing methods available. The same is true for building a social media presence. You and your staff should be promoting your social media accounts at every reasonable opportunity. Whether you mention it in passing or tell a specific patient that you think they would enjoy your content on Facebook, a recommendation directly from a staff member may resonate more than an advertisement on the wall.

Finally, let's consider several forms of Facebook advertising. When used correctly, Facebook ads can be a relatively affordable and effective means for online promotion. I recommend utilizing Facebook ads on three occasions – at your onset or debut, during select recruitment periods or events and from time to time as sponsored or boosted posts. When your Facebook page is just starting out, Facebook advertising makes sense. After you have a solid foundation of friends and family, and your signs, posters and other internal marketing are in place, Facebook advertisements can boost your following among patients. Within your geographic location, some of your patients are surely friends and acquaintances with each other. When you see an advertisement for a Facebook page, Facebook also mentions which of your friends already likes the page. This may prompt other current patients to like your page or spark interest in a new viewer's eyes.

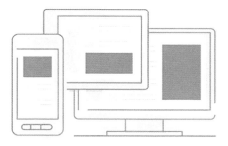

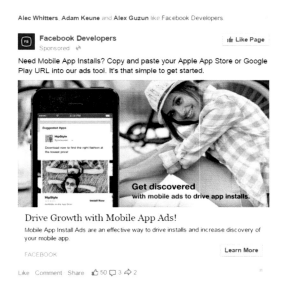

Other campaigns to get more patients to join your page can be supplemented with Facebook advertisements as you see fit. Especially if you are hosting a particular incentive or promotion as a part of your recruitment strategy. This makes the call to action easier to ask for and can be featured on your advertisement or boosted post.

FACEBOOK ADVERTISEMENTS

Here's how Facebook ads work. You pay Facebook to show your advertisement to specific groups of people based on targeting parameters that you can set to designate your intended audience. They are shown on both desktop and mobile platforms. And as more and more people are using their phone, make sure you're creating mobile-friendly ads. Quality, well-targeted ads get more likes, comments and shares, increasing the chances that their friends get to see your ad, compounding your ad's reach. Facebook's "Ads Create Tool" can help you create and optimize your advertisement and the action that you'd like people to take, i.e. engage with your Facebook page, visit your website, claim an offer, etc.

When creating your advertisements, keep several guiding principles in mind. First, consider your target audience. If you're thinking, "I don't have a target, I'll take any patients I can get" I would consider focusing your efforts. It tends to be more effective when you cater to the needs and traits of a certain demographic. For example, even if you would like to target "women" you can consider various subgroups, i.e. college students, new mothers, soccer moms, grandmothers, etc.

Next try to think from the perspective of your target audience. And remember that the general public, of which your patients are members, is not like you. They don't think like you, they don't have your perspective or your humor. So try to relate to them in your advertising. What are *they* like? What do *they* do? What do they find inconvenient and how would your call to action solve this problem? After putting together a proposal, send a screenshot to a few trusted friends or family outside of the dental field and ask them for their opinion.

Also keep in mind one of my favorite mantras – logic makes people think, emotions make people act. Appeal first to emotions, then give a rational reason to make the call or purchase the product or schedule the appointment.

Other markers for successful advertising include being brief and clear in your message. Too much information is no information at all. Is it captivating? Is it memorable? Is it true, honest and authentic? Browse through the next chapter for general characteristics of quality content.

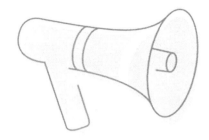

BOOSTED POSTS

"Boosted posts" are a way to increase viewership of specific posts from your page. You can choose to boost the post either at the time you post it or after it has been posted to your page. Boosted posts appear higher in News Feeds, so there's a better chance your audience will see them. You also have a choice of boosting the post to reach a larger percentage of your own fans and their friends or new audiences, all of which can be analyzed through Page Insights. This can be helpful as Facebook started cracking down on posts that appear to be advertisements or overly promotional to limit their reach as of January, 2015. This was implemented in response to several studies showing that users of social media don't appreciate being bombarded with advertisements (duh!). While this limits a business's access to free advertisement, it also forces businesses to create higher quality, more engaging content.

Note that the biggest bang for your buck with boosted posts are posts that you expect to be popular or achieve some form of engagement. This will help spread the message to a considerably larger audience than a simple or mundane advertisement for your practice. Boosting an average post will increase its viewership. Boosting a *quality* post will increase its engagement and send viewership through the roof.

Your highest chance for success is a post that isn't promotional at all, or at least not at first glance. For example, if you've made a charitable donation or if you were featured in the local news, you can post this to your page and boost the post. Don't include your phone number or any sort of "call to action" what so ever. The marketing is implicit in that your face or your name simply appears in the post. It doesn't need to look like an advertisement to act as an advertisement. Contests and giveaways also tend to do well as boosted posts. It's something that you are giving away, and should have no strings attached. Again, the marketing is implied and will go farther than any traditional advertisement touting treatment or services you provide.

FACEBOOK OFFERS

Facebook offers are specific to discounts or promotions that patients can claim and bring into your office. You can boost offers as well to set budgets and target audiences for each offer. If you've ever participated in Groupons or Living Social offers, it is a similar concept but through Facebook.

---

*"Social media is
a team sport."*

4 CHARACTERISTICS OF QUALITY CONTENT

The following is a list of ten characteristics that trend among successful social media posts. While not all-encompassing, these features were compiled through experience, observation and research. You don't need to keep a checklist every time you post, but you should take away guiding principles and put some thought into certain aspects of your content.

1. A VISUAL WITH EVERY POST

Try scrolling through the Facebook news feed on your phone at your usual pace. What catches your attention more, the standard monochromatic font of a text status or the imagery that comes with a picture or video post?

Let's take a look at a screen shot from my news feed on the next page. Even when you first glance at the page, your eyes gravitated towards Dr. Dorfman and his daughter. The AACD wins this round. They shared the news of a member dentist, Dr. Dorfman, who was honored by his alma mater and pictured with his daughter. This post strikes an emotional note regardless of your membership with the AACD. TeleVox for Dentists, on the other hand, featured a "Did you know" post. These educational posts are usually great for small tidbits and fun facts. Unfortunately, TeleVox for Dentist's main audience is dentists, and all of us know that gum disease takes two forms. Still, had the post included a clinical photo or diagram comparing the two forms, this stale statement may have

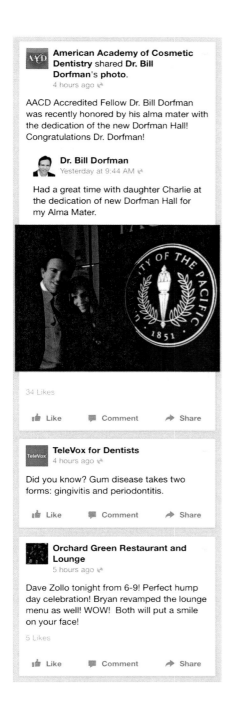

American Academy of Cosmetic Dentistry shared Dr. Bill Dorfman's photo.
4 hours ago

AACD Accredited Fellow Dr. Bill Dorfman was recently honored by his alma mater with the dedication of the new Dorfman Hall! Congratulations Dr. Dorfman!

Dr. Bill Dorfman
Yesterday at 9:44 AM

Had a great time with daughter Charlie at the dedication of new Dorfman Hall for my Alma Mater.

34 Likes

Like   Comment   Share

TeleVox for Dentists
4 hours ago

Did you know? Gum disease takes two forms: gingivitis and periodontitis.

Like   Comment   Share

Orchard Green Restaurant and Lounge
5 hours ago

Dave Zollo tonight from 6-9! Perfect hump day celebration! Bryan revamped the lounge menu as well! WOW! Both will put a smile on your face!

5 Likes

Like   Comment   Share

garnered some engagement. Dentists could have shared the post on their practice page. But instead they likely scrolled right past it because nothing drew your eyes to the post, and even if you read it, you have no reason to interact with it.

This concept is true for any post from any business. To drive the point home, Orchard Green is one of my favorite restaurants back home. They regularly feature a great local artist, Dave Zollo, to perform in the lounge. Zollo has performed there enough times that Orchard Green should have some great shots of Dave playing in the lounge of the restaurant. Patrons that frequent Orchard Green and recognize Dave would have several connections to the news. Anyone unfamiliar with Dave's music may still have recognized the setting of the lounge as a visual cue. Instead, the impression may have been lost altogether with simple text.

People scroll through their phones at a mile a minute. Without an attention-grabbing visual, many posts will simply go unnoticed.

2. BE CONCISE

Your Facebook page may be your stage in a sense, but keep your monologues short. Facebook is a place where short, visual posts work best. Facebook posts should span 1-2 sentences with 1-3 hashtags at most.

If you have a subject you are passionate about, write an original article in your blog. For Facebook, post an attention grabber and then link out to the blog for those interested in reading on. Even blog posts should be kept concise, ideally 1-3 paragraphs with an image or two interspersed throughout. You don't read long, drawn out articles while on Facebook, so don't expect your patients to.

3.   GIVE, GIVE, GIVE, ASK

The Give, Give, Give, Ask concept was formulated by entrepreneur and story-teller Gary Vaynerchuk, who wrote about it in his book *Jab, Jab, Jab, Right Hook*[11] (the name spruces up the concept).

The idea is that businesses on social media tend to engage in two forms of communication with their customers, consumers, clients, etc. The *Give* is simply a conversation piece. It provides small increments of value via a token of information, inspiration, education, entertainment, etc. You are not selling anything or asking for a commitment, you are just sharing a moment together – one engagement at a time that "slowly but authentically builds relationships between brands and customers" as Gary puts it. The *Ask* is the hard sell. It's the action item, e.g. buy our product, subscribe for our services, call our office or schedule an appointment with us.

Gary argues that the most successful way to ask on social media is to give, give, give first (jab, jab, jab). This way, you build leverage for your "ask" (right hook).

This is true for dentists across all social media platforms. If your Facebook posts are full of action items for patients such as "check out our website", "call to schedule an appointment" or "please refer us to a friend" then it should come as no surprise that the posts are overwhelmingly ignored. Instead, the majority of your posts should have no strings attached or ties to scheduling appointments, buying into promotions, etc. You are simply conversing and building a relationship with your patients. In addition to strengthening your bond with current patients, this steady communication will also expedite your bond with new patients, as your social media presence is an expression of the practice's personality, character and values.

4.   BLEND IN

When you log into your personal Facebook account, what do you look for on your News Feed? Are you excited to check out the ads? Hoping to be targeted by big businesses? Probably not. When most people log into Facebook, they are looking for updates from their friends and families, and from a select number of celebrities, brands or local businesses they've chosen to follow. That's what's important to them. For a successful

---

[11] A great read when it comes to social media.

social media relationship, it's critical not to interrupt this experience. Instead, be a part of it. Provide content that looks, sounds, smells and feels exactly like the content they're already looking for. As a general rule, ask yourself – from the standpoint of your audience – would you "like" your own posts?

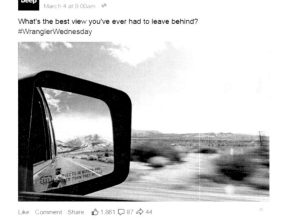

BLENDING IN (AUTHENTIC)

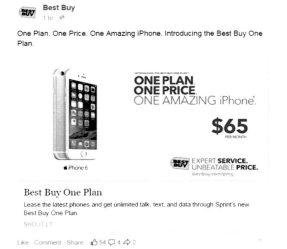

NOT BLENDING IN (ADVERTISEMENT)

5.   HARNESS EMOTIONS

Logic makes people think, emotions make people act. Keep this one in mind. While some facts are interesting on their own, it's hard to "like" an instructional post on dental floss as an average patient. Emotions prompt engagement. Why do cats and dogs rule the internet? They're cute and their antics are hilarious. You can't help but laugh or say "aww" and engage.

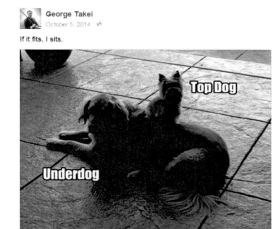

In addition, always add a caption to your photos, whether it's a witty comment or your sincere opinion on the matter. Photos without captions are incomplete thoughts, and people are more likely to respond or join a conversation as opposed to starting their own in the comments section.

6. LEVERAGE POP CULTURE

Is Justin Bieber the poster child for good oral health? Was Batman's uncle a dentist? Does Shrek have perfect teeth? No. But each of these pop culture figures appear on toothbrushes and toothpastes for kids, just like celebrities are used to sell other unrelated products.

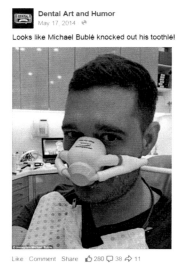

Dental Art and Humor
May 17, 2014

Looks like Michael Bublé knocked out his toothie!

Like Comment Share   280 38 11

You can harness the power of familiarity and pop culture, current events, etc. in a similar fashion. Share articles about celebrities when they chip their front tooth or take selfies at their dental appointments. It's not real news, but it's fun and it relates to your profession. Share your thoughts or comments on various dental headlines or trends. You are the expert and people will want to know your thoughts and opinions on these matters when they come up. Chime in on these conversations!

7. GOOD TIMING

Good marketers know that timing can make or break certain content. If there's a local event or a national news story that relates to teeth, health, dentistry, etc., well-timed delivery can be key.

For a great example of on-the-mark timing, look no further than Snickers. During the 2014 World Cup when Luis Suarez bit another player, a plethora of companies jumped at the opportunity to comment on the event and link it to their product or service. Snickers tweeted "*Hey @luis16suarez. Next time you're hungry just grab a Snickers. #worldcup #luissuarez #EatASNICKERS*" with a clever visual that same day!

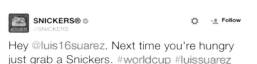

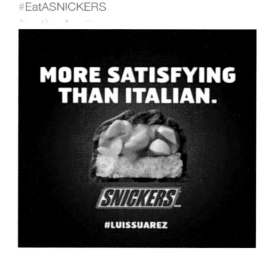

Timing also plays a role with your day-to-day posts. Most people are on

Facebook during the day. If you think of a great photo to post before going to bed, either wait to post it in the morning or schedule it to be posted the day after. Posts will get most of their organic reach within a few hours of their debut. Maximize your potential by posting during the daytime hours of the weekdays and making use of Facebook's "Schedule Post" feature (shown below). You have the ability to see when your specific fans are logging onto Facebook via Insights (discussed in Chapter 7). Scheduled posts also allow your posts to go live during days that your office isn't open so you can "set it and forget it".

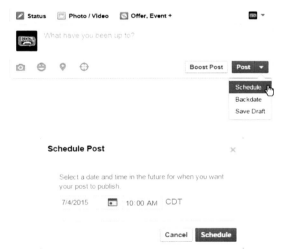

A quick word of caution to keep timing on your side. Facebook allows you to schedule posts months in advance. Keep your scheduled posts in mind in reference to news and world events. For example, if you schedule an upbeat post on a particular topic that happened to make national or tragic news, you want to make sure that doesn't get posted to avoid appearing inappropriate or insensitive. So just keep an eye for your future posts within the context of the times they are set to post.

8.   BE CONSISTENT

Your social media outlets are a means to convey your message. Think about how you'd like to be perceived. In general, you would likely want to convey a welcoming, comforting and relaxed tone with valuable information and light-hearted, family-friendly humor. Make sure every post is consistent with your core values. As the dentist, you should set the tone and make sure you discuss this with any administrator or staff that has the ability to post content to the Facebook page. When there is inconsistency in content, the message is lost.

9.   ATTENTION TO DETAIL

With all of these characteristics, your posts should be well on their way to quality content. But if some of the finer details are overlooked, they may still miss their mark. You wouldn't use dark, pixelated or off-center intraoral photographs for a case presentation, so why post poor-quality images for everyone to see on Facebook? I even see older Docs posting pictures with a dark yellow date and time at the bottom of their grainy photos. This dates you tremendously, and will reflect poorly on how you keep up with the times and technology, especially for today's tech-savvy society. Instead, download a fun photo-editing app that lets you enhance and add designer-quality texts or borders to your photos. They are cheap and relatively easy to use. These small tweaks can really bring photos to life.

10.   CONTEXT IS KEY

Product placement is important. So is context and platform utilization. Although I've mentioned that several social media outlets are looking more and more like Facebook, many have key features and subtle differences that make them unique (see Chapter 8). For this reason, you can't always cut and paste the same content to every site and expect the same results. And while Facebook is still king in terms of its prevalence in the general public, certain demographics are also well represented in the platforms that cater to their preferences, e.g. women on Pinterest. This can play a role when considering your intended audience and which social media platforms you'd like to take part in.

"Social media is an expression of personality, character and values."

5 50 IDEAS FOR YOUR PRACTICE

K eeping in mind that successful posts are short and visual, as well as the other characteristics of quality content mentioned, you are now fully prepared to develop your social media presence.

Many of the items listed in this chapter are recurring dates that can be reused or more appropriately *refreshed* on a yearly basis. Most of them can be easily implemented by your office starting tomorrow. Or better yet... why not today?

Some may be limited by certain aspects of your practice – your building, your location, your staff, the types of procedures you perform, etc. I'll bet you can adapt the unique circumstances of your office to most if not all fifty posts. Be creative. Take the key lessons and components from each post and fit them to meet your needs. Bend the rules. Try new things.

And remember – you and your staff are the most unique and powerful feature of your dental office. Let your personalities shine through, and let's have some fun!

1. Lists

It's only fitting that the first item on our list – is lists. People scroll through their News Feeds at lightening speeds. Take this into account when posting an article you found online or even when writing your own blog content. No patients have the time or interest to read the latest JADA article, but they do have a minute for Huffington Post's "worst foods" or Buzzfeed's celebrity smile makeovers. Lists make information more easily digestible and fun to consume – perfect for social media.

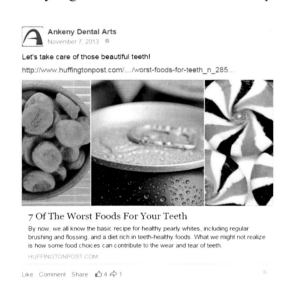

Ankeny Dental Arts
November 7, 2013

Let's take care of those beautiful teeth!

http://www.huffingtonpost.com/.../worst-foods-for-teeth_n_285...

7 Of The Worst Foods For Your Teeth

By now, we all know the basic recipe for healthy pearly whites, including regular brushing and flossing, and a diet rich in teeth-healthy foods. What we might not realize is how some food choices can contribute to the wear and tear of teeth.

HUFFINGTONPOST.COM

Like Comment Share 👍 4 👍 1

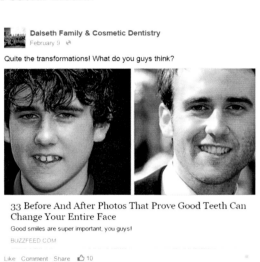

Dalseth Family & Cosmetic Dentistry
February 9

Quite the transformations! What do you guys think?

33 Before And After Photos That Prove Good Teeth Can Change Your Entire Face

Good smiles are super important, you guys!

BUZZFEED.COM

Like Comment Share 👍 10

2. Birthdays

Who doesn't like celebrating their birthday!? Well. Ok. Anyone over 40. But most people at least enjoy celebrating other peoples' birthdays and wishing them well on their special day. Set up a calendar in the break room with everyone's birthday on there – including *yours*. Depending on how many staff are there, that's quite a few posts that write themselves! Even if you don't host a big party for it, every staff member should be wished "Happy Birthday" on Facebook. A picture should always accompany the post, either on their own or with a doctor and the flowers or small gift you got them. And don't forget patients' birthdays! Have a sign or a small gift handy for patients that come in for an appointment on their birthdays.

Waterloo Dental Associates with Christopher Aldrich at **Waterloo Dental Associates**
July 14, 2014

What Dr. Aldrich walked into this morning at the office 😊 Happy 30th!

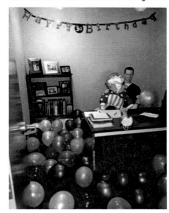

Like   Comment   Share   👍 62 💬 3

Great Florida Smiles & Orthodontics at **Great Florida Smiles & Orthodontics**
February 13

Happy Birthday Dr. MIKE!!!

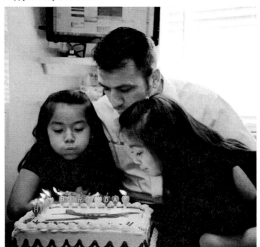

Like   Comment   Share   👍 92 💬 13

Family & Implant Dentistry - Manhattan, Kansas
October 1, 2014

The Best Birthday Wishes going out to this flashy, sassy, fun patient on her 95th Birthday!!! 🎂🍰🎂🍰🎂

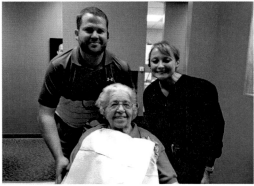

Like   Comment   Share   👍 48 ↪ 1

3. Babies

Everyone loves babies. And eventually, most people *have* babies. It's very relatable content, and if someone in your office has a baby you'd better make a big deal out of it. When the couple brings the baby to the office, snap a picture of them and congratulate them on the newborn!

You can also use this as an educational opportunity to remind other new parents of oral hygiene tips and techniques they can use for their kiddos at home. Take pictures of what you've found to work best when brushing your little guy's teeth.

 The Family Dental Center added 3 new photos.
October 28, 2014 Edited

Emphasis on The FAMILY Dental Center. ☺

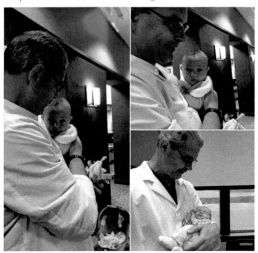

Like   Comment   Share   👍 77 💬 3

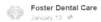 **Foster Dental Care**
January 13

Dr. Foster had a surprise visitor today! He was all smiles for his precious granddaughter.

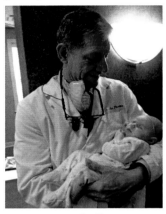

Like   Comment   Share   👍 81 💬 2

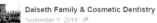 **Dalseth Family & Cosmetic Dentistry**
September 5, 2014

Dr. Jeff and Emily, thanks for coming in today over lunch and showing off Henry. I for one can say he is so darn cute and I loved holding him...Dr. Pascal

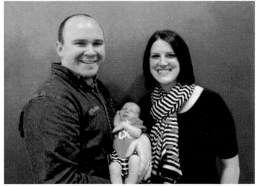

Like   Comment   Share   👍 30 💬 2

4.   Pets

Did someone in the office get a new puppy? Or a fluffy little kitten? Double down on your "aw" factor and share it on your practice's Facebook page. Alternatively, some of your patients may bring their furry friend with them to their appointments. Whether it's for fun or as a service pet, it's unique and you probably don't see that every day. Grab a picture and post how much fun you had sharing your patient's joy with them or thanking their service dog for being such a great companion. Even if you're not crazy about pets, someone in your office can't get enough of them. Let them be in the picture smiling from ear to ear.

Waterloo Dental Associates with Christopher Aldrich
October 16, 2014

Happy Boss's Day Dr. Aldrich!! His puppy Madison decided to pay him a visit. After inspection of her teeth, he instructed her to lay off the sticks.

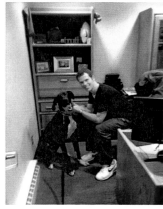

Unlike   Comment   Share   👍 52 💬 5

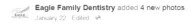

Eagle Family Dentistry added 4 new photos.
January 22   Edited

Happy 1st Birthday to Dr. Dulde's puppy, Cooper! We love you! Cooper says "Hi" to all his friends at the dental office.

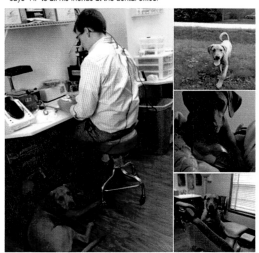

Like   Comment   Share   👍 17 💬 1

Great Florida Smiles & Orthodontics added a new photo to the album: Christmas
December 12, 2014

Dr. Alvarez and his beautiful fiance, Jean, thought posing with their 4 month old puppy would be EASY for a Christmas card! Boy, they were wrong! At least they tried 😊

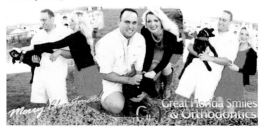

Like   Comment   Share   👍 65 💬 8 ↪ 1

5.   Presents You Give

Are you a generous person? Does your office hold raffles or give out monthly prizes, gift cards and tickets to sporting events? Or maybe the spouse of a hygienist broke their leg and had a hospital stay. Did you bring them flowers or a care package? These are all very marketable practices! Show them off on Facebook!

Great Florida Smiles & Orthodontics
January 30

Another local student that won a $50 gift card from Great Florida Smiles! The winner was excited that the prize was to a book store for she loves to read 😊.

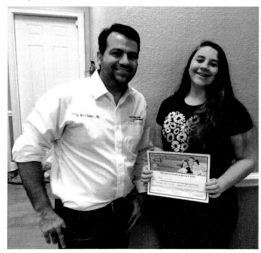

Like   Comment   Share   👍 75 💬 5

2nd Street Dental, LLC with Miranda Haefele and 5 others
May 8, 2014

We took the team to Firerock for a nice lunch and surprised them with the afternoon off and a shopping spree! What a great team and a bunch of fun ladies!

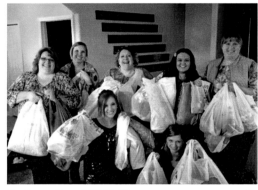

Like   Comment   Share   👍 70 💬 13 ↪ 1

Eagle Family Dentistry at The Garden Mart
May 5, 2014

CONGRATS MICHELLE--winner of $50 gift card to The Garden Mart in Mukwonago! Enjoy planting all of those flowers this week!

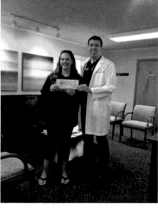

Like   Comment   Share   👍 13

6. Presents You Get

As good as it to give a gift, it's also fun to *get* a gift! Did you get a unique gift from a patient that really appreciated your work? Or did the orthodontist you refer to drop off a pan of brownies? It's ok to show that other people appreciate you as much as you appreciate them. Now, if the orthodontist gave you a Rolex for Christmas, maybe keep that to yourself. Heartfelt gifts, on the other hand, can and should be shared.

Waterloo Dental Associates
December 11, 2014

Cake balls from one of our great specialist! They look too good to eat...but we will 😄

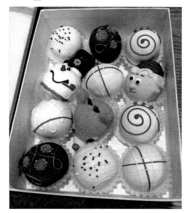

Like Comment Share 👍 26 💬 3

Bondurant Family Dentistry with Steven Neville and Joe
May 20, 2014

Izzy made Dr Neville a necklace today!

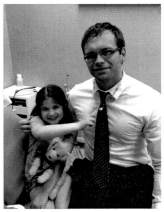

Like Comment Share 👍 97 💬 9

East County Endodontics
January 14, 2014

Past patient Frederick brought our team "good fortune" in the form of cookies today! Thank you Frederick!

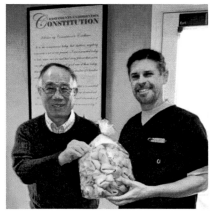

Like Comment Share 👍 31 💬 1

7.   Staff Profiles & New Hires

Staff profiles are a great way for your Facebook fans to get to know you and your staff, especially new hires. Similar to your staff profiles on your website, staff profiles on social media can be a running theme that can fill a slow week or be tacked onto another post such as someone's birthday. Feature fun information including questionnaires, hidden talents, pets, etc.

This can be a serious relationship builder for new and existing patients. Let's say a long time patient of yours is hoping to get a cleaning in before leaving on a trip to Madrid with her husband. On her News Feed pops up a profile of your newest hygienist whose favorite travel destination is listed as Spain. Think she'll make a request to fill an open spot with the new hygienist? You bet! Or let's say a new patient just moved into town from Michigan where she just finished a graduate program. While browsing a few dentists in the area she checks out your Facebook page to see that your receptionist's favorite sports team is the Wolverines. Your practice will feel like home as soon as walks in the front door!

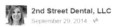

2nd Street Dental, LLC
September 29, 2014

We would like to give a warm welcome to our new dental assistant, Cherie! We are thrilled for you to join our team at 2nd Street Dental!

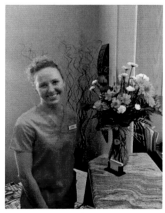

Like   Comment   Share   👍 35   💬 4

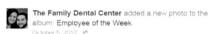

The Family Dental Center added a new photo to the album: Employee of the Week.
October 5, 2012

MEET JoLynn!

I am a dental hygienist at The Family Dental Center! I also educate patients about their dental health. I have been in the dental hygiene field for six years and have worked for 3 years at The Family Dental Center.
I enjoy spending time with my family and friends. I like running, watching Hawkeye football, gardening, and traveling.
My favorite thing about working at The Family Dental Center is that we are one big family and we help take care of each other as w... See More

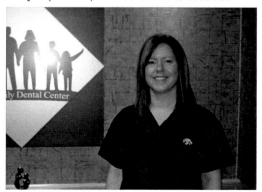

Like   Comment   Share   👍 12

8.   Office Tour & Photos

An album featuring photos of your office is an essential component of both your website and your Facebook page. I strongly suggest having professional photos taken by someone who has some experience with real estate photography. The iPhone has come a long way, but the results just won't be the same. They'll set the stage, get the lighting right and take your practice from good to great. While your pride rests on the shoulders of your best dental work, the physical space of your office is of utmost importance to patients. It's a means of building familiarity and comfort, and patients will make assumptions based on the cleanliness and atmosphere of your dental practice.

"But what if my building isn't particularly grand or inspiring?"

Your photographer can help, and so can you. Maybe your practice is in a strip mall, so the outside of your building isn't its greatest asset. Build character on the inside and liven up the space with unique style and decor. Is there a park or attraction nearby? Take a candid photo on the walk you took after work one day. Express how nice it is that this place or other attractions are close by to your office. Does your office back up to a wooded area? Snap a photo of the deer through your window. Even a particularly nice sunset taken from your office can make for a pleasant post from time to time.

Ivory Dental Group added 3 new photos
August 26, 2014

Photos of our new space!

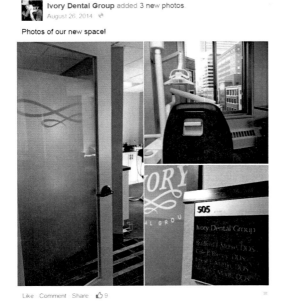

Like Comment Share 👍 9

Eagle Family Dentistry updated their cover photo.
January 7

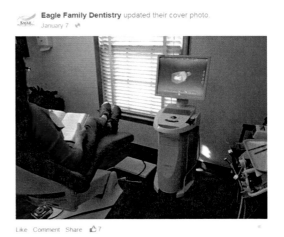

Like Comment Share 👍 7

9. Technology

Patients tend to associate the newest and hottest technology with high quality dentistry. While we know that's not necessarily true, can we blame them? We're attracted to new phones, cars, shiny things, etc. If you're going digital with x-rays, CAD-CAM, anything... flaunt it! Take a picture of the machine being installed and thank the company that installs it. Take a picture of the final product and briefly explain how it will benefit *the patient.* Don't focus on the minute details or specifications, instead focus on how it will help you provide better treatment or the features that will make for a more pleasant patient experience. For example, don't tout the resolution and micron-accuracy of your new Cerec scanner, instead show how patients will no longer have to deal with that nasty, goopy impression material!

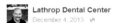

Lathrop Dental Center
December 4, 2013

Our 3D x-ray unit is being installed. This will allow us to see everything in the mouth in 3D. Very important for placing dental implants and oral surgery. Less than 1% of dental offices have this technology in office. We are proud to offer the most advanced technology available.

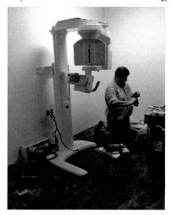

Like Comment Share 👍 34

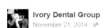

Ivory Dental Group
November 21, 2014

Our Newest Ivory Dental Addition: Watch Netflix instead of Stare at Ceiling Tiles!!!

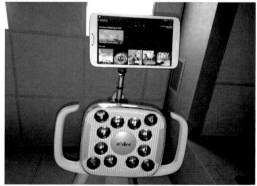

Unlike Comment Share 👍 25 💬 1

10.   Work Anniversaries

I'm referencing work anniversaries, but the milestone personal anniversaries can also be shared on Facebook. It not only thanks the staff members that have been with you through the years but it also signals to patients that your office must be a great place to work for someone. Celebrate and thank your employees with flowers or another small token of your appreciation. Again, a heads up that their picture may be taken is usually appreciated.

Dalseth Family & Cosmetic Dentistry added 3 new photos.
June 5, 2014

Congratulations Yvonne on your 15 year anniversary here at Dalseth Family and Cosmetic Dentistry. You have been a great team member and an outstanding hygienist. All of us, including our patients appreciate all you do. Thank you!

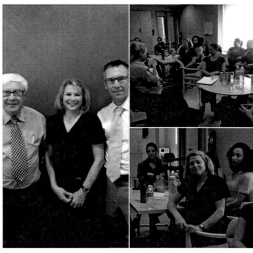

Like   Comment   Share   👍 28 💬 7

Bondurant Family Dentistry with Steven Neville and 3 others
June 3, 2014

She's been Bondurant's finest hygienist for 1 year today folks! Fantastic!

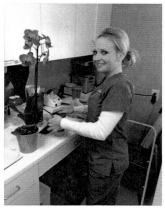

Like   Comment   Share   👍 82 💬 4

2nd Street Dental, LLC
November 19, 2014

Thank you and congratulations to our front office guru, Sam, on her 2 years of service at 2nd Street Dental! Click like if you enjoy seeing Sam's friendly face when you walk in our door.

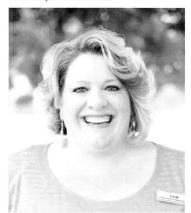

Like   Comment   Share   👍 47 💬 8 ↗ 1

11. Practice Anniversaries

If your practice doors have been open for 5 years – celebrate! 10 years? 20? 35? Even better! Whether it's every year or the milestone years, put up a Facebook post with an authentic and heartfelt caption. Reflect on the years and how much you've truly enjoyed being able to provide the care that you do. Thank your patients and the community.

Broadhollow Dentistry
February 22, 2014

Today is our 4 year anniversary! Thank you to all of our amazing patients for making our office a fun place to be.

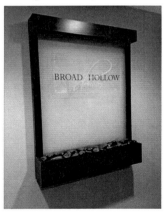

Like   Comment   Share   👍 65 💬 3

Bondurant Family Dentistry with Steven Neville and 3 others
February 8, 2014

Celebrating 2 years of Bondurant Family Dentistry! Thank you for being a part of our success!

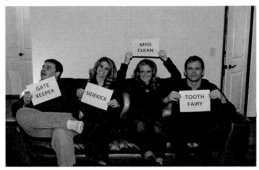

Like   Comment   Share   👍 170 💬 12 ↪ 1

Marshalltown Family Dentistry added 2 new photos — hnson.
May 20, 2014

One year ago today was our first day as Marshalltown Family Dentistry! The staff surprised us with cake and a potluck. Here's to many, many more! Thanks to all our patients for sticking with us!

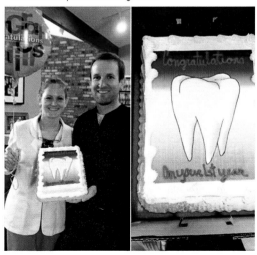

Like   Comment   Share   👍 19 💬 2 ↪ 1

12.   Continuing Education

Continuing education is mandatory for you as a clinician. It improves your techniques and keeps you up-to-date with the latest and greatest in dentistry. It also benefits your patients, but do they know that you took that course on complex endodontics last month? Or that you recently went to the state dental meeting with your entire staff and had a blast seeing old friends and colleagues?

Get photos at every event and "Check In" at the venue to give your patients a real-time backstage pass to the educational commitment you've made. If part or all of your team joins you, make sure you have someone snap a group photo! If the hosts of the CE are savvy, they may even be one step ahead of you. Some events have a professional photographer on site with fun props and signs for group photos as a courtesy to those that participate.

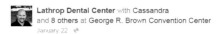

Lathrop Dental Center with Cassandra and 8 others at George R. Brown Convention Center
January 22

Getting our continuing education on at The Star of the South Conference

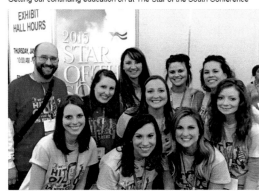

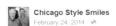

Like   Comment   Share   👍 28   💬 3

Chicago Style Smiles
February 24, 2014

Chicago's annual Dental Midwinter was last weekend, this is a dental conference where dentists from around the world learn about new products and take class. While checking out Colgate's new products look who Dr. Dow ran into, his childhood super hero Donatello!

http://www.cds.org/Midwinter_Meeting/Midwinter_Meeting.aspx

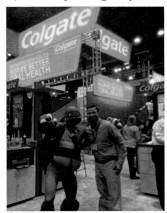

Like   Comment   Share   👍 14

13. Dental Tips & Educational Posts

You may have an educational blog connected to your website. You can and should share the links to these posts on your social media outlets. However, rarely does anyone other than Google "read" those articles. Most dentists keep a running blog simply for its SEO (search engine optimization) benefits.

When it comes to patient engagement, educational posts for social media are very different and actually more effective. Include a relevant picture. Keep it short and to-the-point – one or two sentences at most. Scrolling through news feeds doesn't allow much time for your sermon on proper flossing technique. Don't expect much interaction with these posts, but do include them in your social media collection, as it shows commitment to your profession and education. Plus, you're a dentist. Some dental gospel is expected and acceptable.

Orange City Dentistry
February 19, 2014

Wednesday Whitening Tip:

Did you know that any food or drink that will stain a white t-shirt, can also stain your teeth? Drinks like coffee, dark colored pop, fruit juice, sports drinks, and red wine will stain your teeth. Be like Princess Kate, try drinking these beverages through a straw!

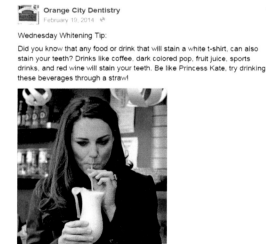

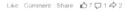
Like Comment Share 👍 7 💬 1 ↪ 2

Consamus and Hampton Dental
January 17, 2014

Fun fact for your Friday! Sugar-less chewing gum can be helpful for your teeth, especially after a meal! #funfact

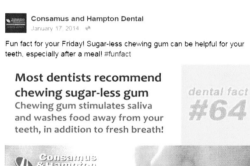

Most dentists recommend chewing sugar-less gum
Chewing gum stimulates saliva and washes food away from your teeth, in addition to fresh breath!

dental fact **#64**

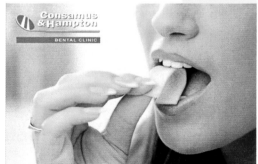

Like Comment Share 👍 4

14. The Weather & All Four Seasons

Seasons are four freebies that you can count on every year. Whether you're saying goodbye to the old or welcoming the new season, find a fitting photograph and type up your two cents about the change. Make your best guess at the forecast. Or what kind of weather are you hoping for? Compare this year's winter to last year's winter. And if you practice in San Diego, make light of the fact that you won't really be having a winter, just like last year and the year before that!

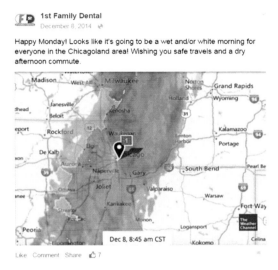

1st Family Dental
December 8, 2014

Happy Monday! Looks like it's going to be a wet and/or white morning for everyone in the Chicagoland area! Wishing you safe travels and a dry afternoon commute.

Dec 8, 8:45 am CST

Like Comment Share 👍 7

2nd Street Dental, LLC
March 20, 2014

Happy Spring!

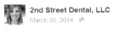
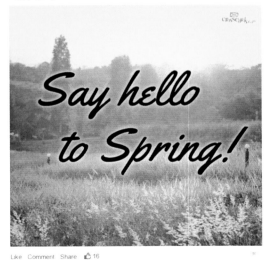

Like Comment Share 👍 16

Watertown Dental Care
January 5, 2014

Stay Warm Everyone!

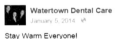
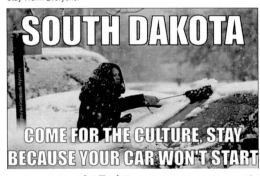

Like Comment Share 👍 17 💬 1 ↗ 16

15. Inspirational Quotes & Motivational Monday

It's safe to say that most working individuals dread Mondays. Even if you do too, I wouldn't recommend joining the Debbie Downers of the world and complaining about it. Instead, I'd use Monday (or any day for that matter) as an opportunity to be uplifting and inspiring. It may be a touch cliché, but who doesn't love a great quote once in a while? And I'm not talking about cutting and pasting a quote into the status bar of your page. I'm talking about a picture of a historical figure or a great landscape with a bold quote above the horizon. If you take the photo yourself, throw in your logo or practice name in the corner using Photoshop or a photo-editing app.

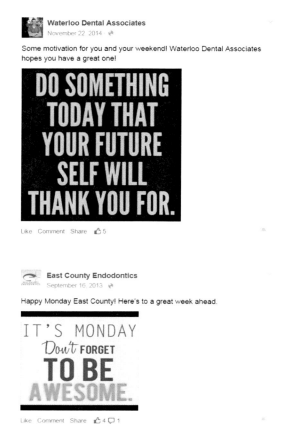

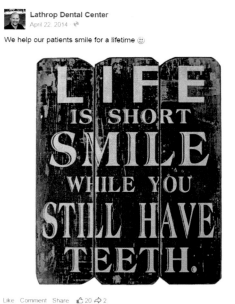

16. Throwback Thursday

Throwback Thursday is a social media trend that is denoted by the hashtag #TBT. On any given Thursday, you reminisce about anything during any time in history. People usually share old photographs of themselves. Companies and brands share photos from their early years or the history of their industry. Dentists can post their class photos from dental school, old photos of the practice or outdated technologies, vintage dental advertisements, etc. Or try featuring a "guess who" or mix and match with old staff photos. Make sure to tag it with #TBT. Or for those that can't get enough of the throwbacks, #FBF (Flashback Friday).

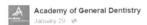

Academy of General Dentistry
January 29

Blast from the past! The AGD's Executive Committee at our Annual Meeting in Chicago '75 #TBT

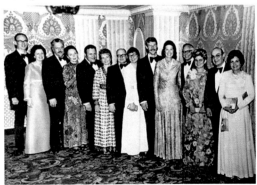

Like   Comment   Share   👍 32   💬 5

Family & Implant Dentistry - Manhattan, Kansas
November 7, 2013

Its time for another #throwbackthursday!

Once a team always a team! Mark has been passing his skills down since Rawley was just a wee one.... I wonder if they are as good at fishing as they are at dentistry??

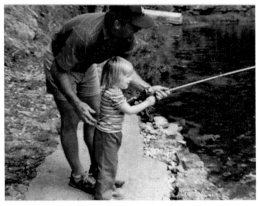

Like   Comment   Share   👍 31

Orange City Dentistry
August 26 at 7:06am

For your back to school outfit, don't forget to wear your smile! Here's Dr. Mark showing how it's done on his way to 1st grade.

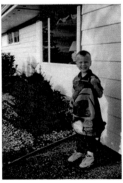

Like   Comment   Share   👍 45   💬 4

17.   Fridays

Little brings more joy to people every week than Friday. It's a universal celebration for the working class. If you don't work on Fridays, don't post your view from the golf course. Instead, schedule a post with a funny comic (#FridayFunny) or a fun fact or anything that can be related to the joy and relief that Friday tends to bring. Tons of "Happy Friday" content is spread all across the internet every week. Share it and rejoice with your patients!

Waterloo Dental Associates
April 10

Hmmm, now that's optimism 😊 Happy Friday!

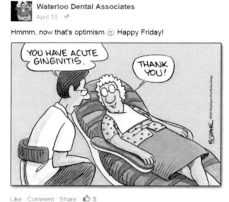

Like Comment Share 👍 5

1st Family Dental
July 23 at 2:32pm

Smile! It's almost Friday. 😊

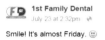
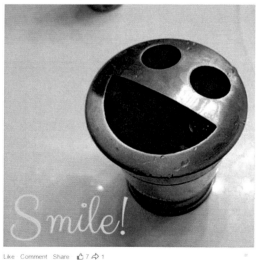

Like Comment Share 👍 7 ↗ 1

Lathrop Dental Center
September 12 2014

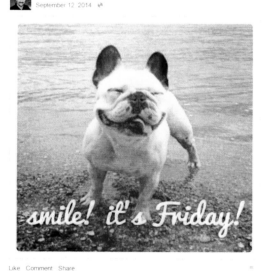

Like Comment Share

18. Internet Trends

Some internet trends are worth getting into. For example, how many of your friends were nominated for the Polar Plunge? Or the ALS Ice Bucket Challenge? It was fun, interactive and helped support a great cause. Some practices were nominated as a whole, and for some it was an excuse for staff to dump a bucket of ice cold water on their boss! Stay in tune with internet trends and if it works for your practice, get in on the fun!

Dr. Michael Hopkins Dental Office
August 19, 2014

Dr. Hopkins has been challenged by Lynn Atkinson for the #ALS #icebucket challenge! Please visit http://www.alsa.org/donate/ to make a donation today!

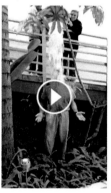

Like   Comment   Share   👍 92   💬 7

Orange City Dentistry
April 19, 2014

Watch Dr. Mark take the plunge for Landon! Thanks Glen Bonnema for the nomination.

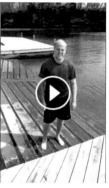

Unlike   Comment   Share   👍 21   💬 6

Family & Implant Dentistry - Manhattan, Kansas
August 25, 2014 · Edited

Thanks Tindall Orthodontics for the nomination!!! Each like this video gets the docs have agreed to donate $1 extra to the ALS Foundation!!

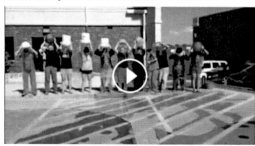

Like   Comment   Share   👍 700   💬 6   ↪ 31

19.   All Major Holidays

Take advantage of these special days that are conveniently scattered throughout the year as a way to keep in touch with your patients. Wish them a "Happy Labor Day". Wear green for St. Patrick's Day. Pull up one of your favorite Martin Luther King Jr quotes. Have a post for *every* official holiday. A list of all major holidays can be found in Chapter 6.

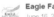 **Eagle Family Dentistry** added 3 new photos
June 16, 2014 · Edited ·

Dad---Happy Father's Day and thanks for everything you do to support Eagle Family Dentistry!

My dad is officially the first patient I saw in private practice. He's also a great mentor, business coach, friend, and a tireless volunteer around the office. You're the best dad a dentist could ask for!

-Dr. Dulde

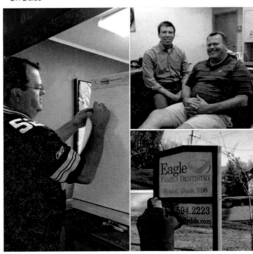

Like   Comment   Share   👍 29

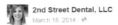 **2nd Street Dental, LLC**
March 18, 2014 ·

We made sure not to get pinched! Did anyone else have a fun St. Patty's Day yesterday?!

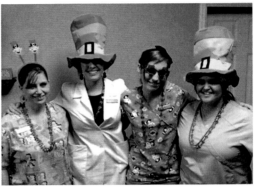

Like   Comment   Share   👍 35

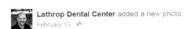 **Lathrop Dental Center** added a new photo.
February 13 ·

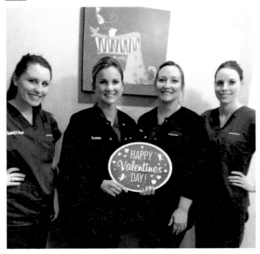

Like   Comment   Share   👍 22 💬 1

20. Unofficial Holidays & Commemorative Dates

We may not get the day off from work for National Puppy Day (March 23rd), Star Wars Day (May 4th) or Left Handers Day (August 13th). But that doesn't mean you can't take advantage of these fun days! You can Google "unofficial holidays list" or find your favorite unofficial holidays from a number of sources.

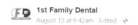

1st Family Dental
August 13 at 9:42am · Edited ·

Happy #lefthanders Day! Cheers to our left-handed staff & dental professionals, and to the dental assistants who can reverse everything they do for our lefties without batting an eye. 😊

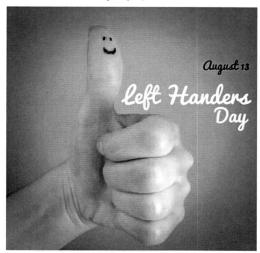

Like Comment Share 👍 22 💬 2 ↪ 2

East County Endodontics
March 23 ·

Dr. Hornberger and Halo. Happy National Puppy Day!

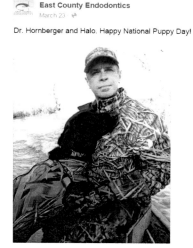

Like Comment Share 👍 31 💬 2

Dr. Michael Hopkins Dental Office with Michael Hopkins and 4 others
April 2, 2014 ·

Each year 1 in 68 kids are impacted by Autism. Today we proudly wore blue to raise awareness and support for World Autism Awareness Day and Light It Up Blue! #LIUB #AutismAwareness

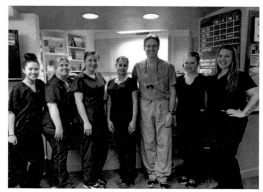

Like Comment Share 👍 59 💬 5

21. Halloween

While I recommend all holidays have a Facebook post to accompany them, some holidays are special enough to get their own headline.

Does your practice dress up for Halloween? Do you encourage patients to dress up? You should!

Halloween is a versatile holiday. Try hosting a Facebook contest for "Best Costume" within your staff, or even your patients. Have a staff member make a numbered collage. Whoever has the most likes or comments with their number wins a prize. Grab a picture of the winner with his or her prize for another post in two or three days while Halloween is still in mind.

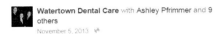

Halloween Dress Up at Watertown Dental Care!

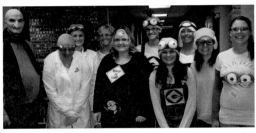

Like Comment Share 👍 62 💬 5

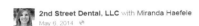

We had a surprise visit from Spider-Man today! ☺

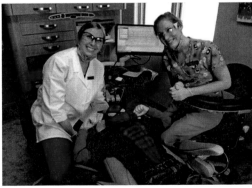

Like Comment Share 👍 39 💬 2 ↪ 1

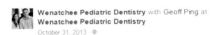

Dr Maverick and Dr Batman here to save the day!

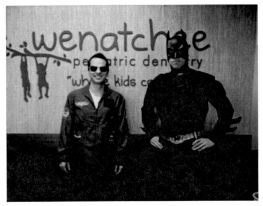

Like Comment Share 👍 517 💬 18

22.   Halloween Candy Buy-Back

"Halloween Candy Buy-Back" is another big hit around this time of year. The idea is to either accept drop-offs or buy back candy from the community for $1 or $2 per pound. Several weeks prior, you can register your practice at www.halloweencandybuyback.com. Collections are then sent to deployed troops through Operation Gratitude or other military organizations.

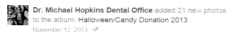

Dr. Michael Hopkins Dental Office added 21 new photos to the album: Halloween/Candy Donation 2013.
November 12, 2013

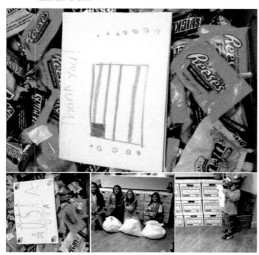

Like Comment Share 👍 16

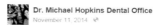

Dr. Michael Hopkins Dental Office
November 11, 2014

Thank you to everyone who took the time to collect and drop off their unwanted candy! This year was a great success, we collected over 700 lbs of candy to send to Afghanistan for the troops! #supportthetroops #operationgratitude

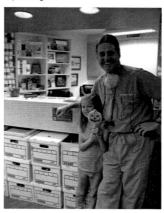

Like Comment Share 👍 289 💬 4 ↪ 1

Scott Adishian, D.D.S., Inc.
January 21, 2014

At Scott Adishian, D.D.S., Inc.

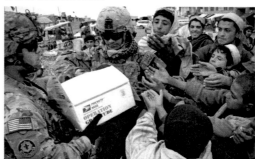

Like Comment Share

23. Veteran's Day & Military Care Packages

Chances are, a staff member or family/friend of a staff member is or was in the military. Veterans Day is special because it celebrates unsung heroes, some of whom we are lucky enough to have contact with. Feature and thank these veterans for their service.

Sending a care package to a military member abroad or at home is also a great way to boost moral both for the soldier and the office. Have everyone in the office sign the card with the aid. Not sure what to send? There are plenty of articles out there. *"What Deployed Troops Really Want in Their Care Packages"* by Jonathan Pharr is a good place to start. And the comments section is full of stories from readers. Even if you don't know any deployed troops directly, there are programs out there that can link you to the troops. For example, *Adopt A US Soldier* (www.adoptaussoldier.org) is a non-profit that connects supportive civilians with our troops overseas.

Marshalltown Family Dentistry
November 11, 2014

Happy Veteran's Day and THANK YOU to all the men and women who serve our country and sacrifice for our freedom. Can you pick out Dr. Dan?

"This nation will remain the land of the free only so long as it is the home of the brave." – Elmer Davis

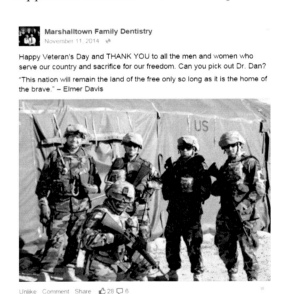

Unlike Comment Share 👍 28 💬 6

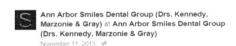

Ann Arbor Smiles Dental Group (Drs. Kennedy, Marzonie & Gray) at Ann Arbor Smiles Dental Group (Drs. Kennedy, Marzonie & Gray)
November 11, 2013

Thank You to all of our veterans, especially Amy Redente and Lorenzo Banda, who work so hard to make Ann Arbor Smiles Dental Group (Drs. Kennedy, Marzonie & Gray) an even better place!

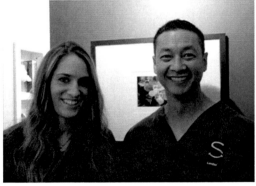

Like Comment Share 👍 23 💬 1

24.   Elf on the Shelf

As soon as Halloween's over with and Thanksgiving dinner is down the hatch, what do all businesses gravitate towards? The winter holiday season, Christmas and the gang. As soon as you start to feel the holiday spirit, usually during the first few weeks of December, order yourself a small action figure known as *Elf on the Shelf.* Make it a holiday tradition to name the little guy (or girl) and place him (or her) in various scenes having little adventures around the office. It's cute. It's fun. It's marketable.

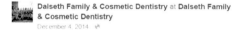

Dalseth Family & Cosmetic Dentistry at Dalseth Family & Cosmetic Dentistry
December 4, 2014

Looks like we got a special delivery today! Only problem is this little #elf doesn't have a name yet... any suggestions???

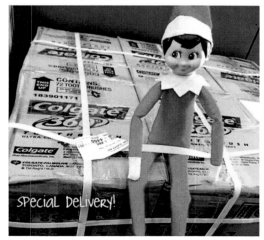

SPECIAL DELIVERY!

Unlike Comment Share   👍 11 💬 7

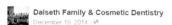

Dalseth Family & Cosmetic Dentistry
December 19, 2014

Like Dr Pascal, Flossie craves adventure! Here he is zip-lining with some floss on the indoor terrain of our front desk! #FlossieTheElf

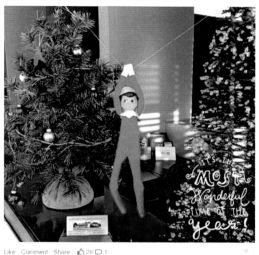

Like Comment Share   👍 28 💬 1

Family & Implant Dentistry - Manhattan, Kansas
December 23, 2014

Bruxzir is pickin' up the ladies in this place!! 😊😊

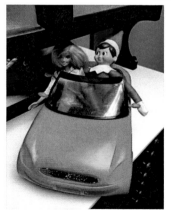

Like Comment Share   👍 18

25. Christmas

Does your office do anything special for the winter holidays? It should! Winter is tough enough as it is. We could all use a little Christmas cheer. Put up holiday decorations. Have a gift exchange and wear ugly sweaters. Heck, have the senior dentist dress up like Santa! Or have a gingerbread house competition with your team and have your patients vote for their favorite one. Post a picture of the cookies you left for Santa. The possibilities are endless! And keep in mind you can still wish everyone a Merry Christmas even if you do not personally celebrate Christmas. The same is true for other holidays. Be sure to have a post for Hanukkah and Kwanzaa too!

 Waterloo Dental Associates with Christopher Aldrich and 8 others
December 18, 2014

A very merry Christmas and happy holidays from WDA! We are so thankful to have each other and our patients! We wish you all smiles and love over the season!

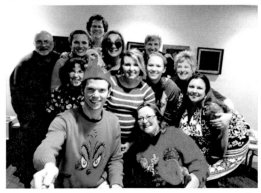

Unlike Comment Share 👍 78 💬 13

 Bondurant Family Dentistry with Steven Neville and 3 others
December 23, 2013

Comment and tell us who has the best holiday sweater. Winner gets dinner from the other 3! Happy Holidays and Happy New Year!

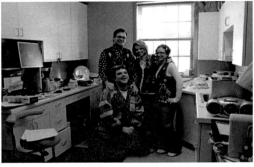

Like Comment Share 👍 52 💬 54

 Foster Dental Care added 53 new photos to the album: Santa at Foster Dental Care — at **Foster Dental Care**
December 9, 2014

For the second year in a row, Santa Claus has come to Foster Dental Care to take pictures with patients of all ages. Our office is full of cheer and smiles!

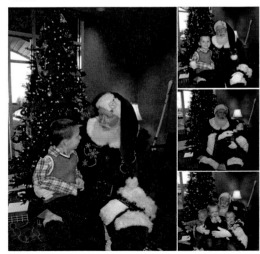

Like Comment Share 👍 25

26.   Office Parties

There's no shame in getting together for a little office fun – outside the office. In fact, it's great for morale and team building, and it's great to share some of the goofiness that comes out when a group of people are having fun. Whether it's at the doctor's house, your favorite restaurant or if your team gets together for a few rounds of bowling, patients like to see that the team gets together to celebrate birthdays, holidays, local events or even a wine tasting (just snap the photos before anyone's eyes get too heavy).

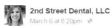
2nd Street Dental, LLC
March 6 at 6:20pm

The smiles say it all in this photo! We had a great time relaxing and painting after a busy work week. Kalah wasn't able to be there and we all missed her presence!

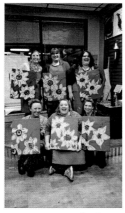

Like Comment Share 👍 28 💬 7

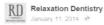
Relaxation Dentistry
January 11, 2014

At the Brunswick zone in Eden prairie for our holiday party!

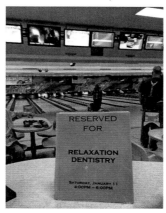

Like Comment Share 👍 7 💬 1

Waterloo Dental Associates with Christopher Aldrich and 5 others
March 21, 2014

Waterloo Dental Associate's staff and spouses enjoyed a fun Mexican fiesta together! And the night included a surprise "puppy shower" for Dr. Aldrich's new pup, Madison!

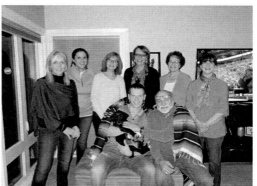

Like Comment Share 👍 30 💬 3

27. Marathons, 5K's and Fun Runs

Your team may not be passing any batons in the next Olympic Games. And that's ok. The runs I'm referring to are the local 5K's and 10K's that can be walked or ran to help support various organizations. These small races are great team-building exercises. Add some fun to the mix by having a team name and matching shirts for your staff and any of their spouses or family members participating in the race. This not only helps your staff find each other at the end but it's free marketing both at the event and on social media.

If someone in your office is in fact an athlete that completes half or whole marathons, make sure to cheer them on and have them post a picture or two from the event. These races require months of disciplined training and the inspiring atmosphere at a big race can be a fun way to spend a Saturday or Sunday morning. You can even help sponsor these types of events to really get your name out there!

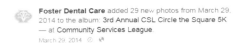

Foster Dental Care added 29 new photos from March 29, 2014 to the album: 3rd Annual CSL Circle the Square 5K — at Community Services League.
March 29, 2014

For the 3rd year in a row, Foster Dental Care sponsored the Circle the Square 5K, benefiting the Community Services League. We paid the race fee for 50 patients and had a great time running/walking for an amazing cause. See you all next year! (thank you seeKCrun.com for the great pictures)

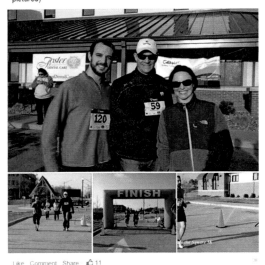

Like Comment Share 👍 11

Marshalltown Family Dentistry
May 31, 2014

Happy Birthday to Dr. Mikki! These two celebrated by doing the Dam to Dam half marathon, where she showed Dr. Dan a thing or two about running :)

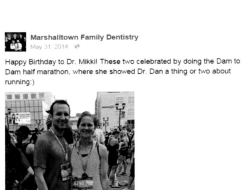

Like Comment Share 👍 15 💬 1 ↪ 2

28. Volunteering

Does your practice as a whole or individually volunteer their time at least once a year for any event, dental or otherwise? Consider doing this not only as a team function but also as a service to those in need. Patients will be delighted to know that you are giving back and staying involved with your community. If you're wondering where to get started, consider a Mission of Mercy or getting in touch with your local rotary club.

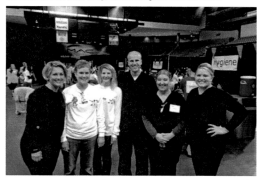

Orange City Dentistry
September 11

We had a great day at Iowa Mission of Mercy helping hundreds of people receive free extractions, fillings and cleanings for healthier smiles!

Like   Comment   Share   👍 28   ↩ 1

Dalseth Family & Cosmetic Dentistry added 13 new photos to the album: Friday afternoon at Feed My Starving Children — at Feed My Starving Children.
September 21, 2013

We had a great afternoon packing meals to be shipped to Haiti. We all looked our best with our fancy hair nets as we packed 10584 meals.

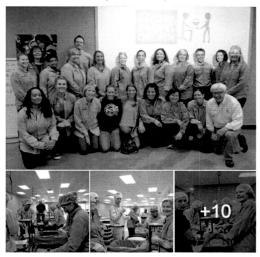

Like   Comment   Share   👍 18

Flucke & Associates Dentistry added 2 new photos.
July 17, 2014

We took an afternoon this week to volunteer at Harvesters. Harvesters feeds 66,000 people a week. Incredible.

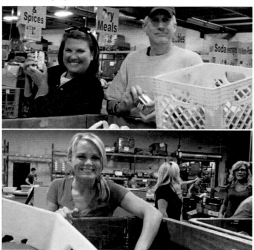

Like   Comment   Share   👍 21   💬 4

29. Before & After Photos

Dentistry is your craft. If you provide quality work there's nothing wrong with showcasing it from time to time. Obviously posting a before/after of an extraction isn't what we're talking about (now you see it, now you don't!). Your esthetic dentistry, on the other hand, is very, very marketable.

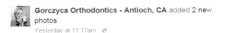

Gorczyca Orthodontics - Antioch, CA added 2 new photos.
Yesterday at 11:17am

"Braces were the best thing that ever happened to me!"

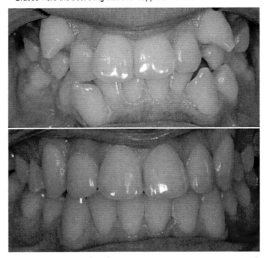

Like Comment Share 👍 10 ↪ 3

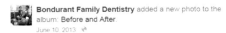

Bondurant Family Dentistry added a new photo to the album: Before and After.
June 10, 2013

Accidents can happen on a Sunday. All fixed up and ready for work on Monday!

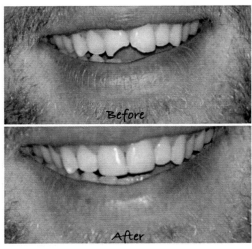

Like Comment Share 👍 55 💬 5

Make your pictures clean and presentable, no blood and guts or mid-treatment photos. The chipped tooth, the smile before and after veneers, the dentures that changed someone's life. That's what patients can clearly see and relate to, and that's where the gold is. You'll have to get your patient's permission, and if they don't want a full-face shot, you'll have to make do with the up-close ones. But you'll find that many patients are accepting and don't mind having their picture taken, especially when they're happy with the results!

30.   Social Signs

Social signs are a fun way for patients and staff to get involved with your social media activity. Essentially, social signs are short words, phrases or images printed and laminated on quality paper. They can be used for almost any and all occasions, from birthdays and holidays to sports teams and contests. Just hold up the sign, smile and post it to your social accounts.

Simple. Easy. Effective. Not sure where to start? Email me. I'm a nerd about this stuff!

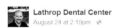

Lathrop Dental Center
August 24 at 2:19pm

Have a wonderful First Day of school, hoping all the kids are wearing their smiles
#LDC #FirstdayofSchool #HappymommysandDaddys

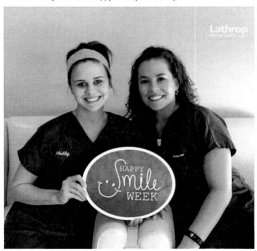

Like   Comment   Share   👍 40 💬 3

Gorczyca Orthodontics - Antioch, CA
July 9, 2014

Welcome to our summer intern Ebony. Ebony has applied to dental school and has wanted to be an orthodontist since she was 9 years old! Great to have you with us!

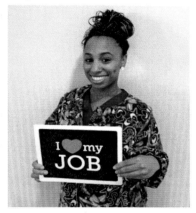

Like   Comment   Share   👍 31 💬 2

Family & Implant Dentistry - Manhattan, Kansas
November 1, 2013

Happy Friday!!!
Now let's hear how many of you love your dentist? (Never mind our cute photobomber) #tgif #photobomb #I♥Mydentist

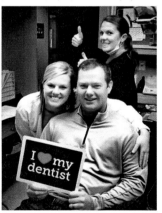

Like   Comment   Share   👍 36 💬 2

31. Celebrity Smiles

Celebrity Smiles can be a fun game and a running segment on your wall. The way it works is that you crop a photo of a well-known celebrity's smile, and ask people to guess which celebrity owns those pearly whites. Don't make it too tricky at first. Later that day or the next day, you can respond in the comments section with the complete picture of the celebrity's face and the answer. Pride points or small gifts for the winners at their next dental visit!

Consamus and Hampton Dental
December 11, 2013

It's time for another edition of CELEBRITY SMILES! We think you "will" have no problem guessing this one! Any takers?

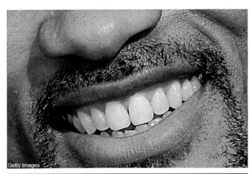

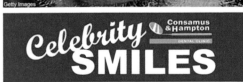

Like Comment Share 👍 3 💬 5

Dalseth Family & Cosmetic Dentistry
February 4

It's time for another edition of Celebrity Smiles! Can you put a name this newlywed's teeth?

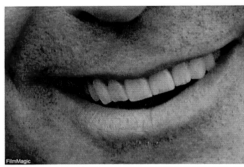

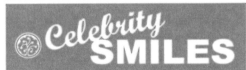

Like Comment Share 👍 2 💬 5

Answer:

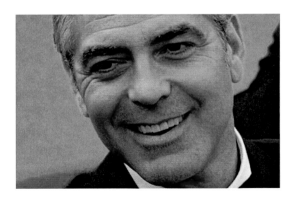

32. Comics & Memes

Comics and memes are perfect for social media. For those unfamiliar, a meme is simply a photo with a bold white caption stamped onto the top or bottom of an image. They're usually fun, playful and easily digestible information. You can even make your own with one of many meme generators, and it doesn't always have to be a dental cartoon or meme. It can be a good one about the weather, Fridays, puns, etc. It's important to keep your humor in check by keeping it PG, and stay well away from hot-button topics such as politics or religion.

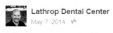

Lathrop Dental Center
May 7, 2014

Office Space never gets old

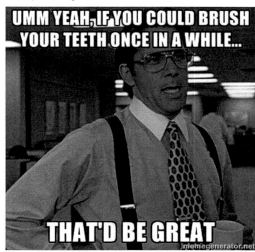

Like Comment Share 👍 18

Consamus and Hampton Dental
December 23, 2013

Careful what you say over the holidays! 😊

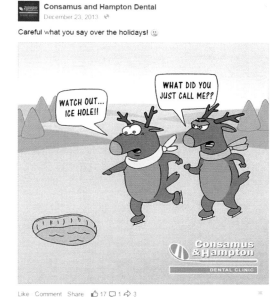

Like Comment Share 👍 17 💬 1 ↪ 3

Howard Farran DDS, MBA
October 13, 2014

Me and my dental chair... We go way back!

#DentalPuns #DentalHumor #DentalJokes

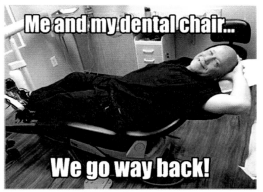

Like Comment Share 👍 708 💬 21 ↪ 20

33.   April Fools & Office Pranks

Any pranksters in your office? April Fools is a fun excuse for office pranks... but just about any day will do! Think along the lines of the friendly feud between Jim Halpert and Dwight Schrute on *The Office*. If you can capture a good, clean practical joke on camera (photo or video), share it on your page.

 Waterloo Dental Associates shared Annie's video.
May 6, 2014

A practical joke played on Dr. Christopher Aldrich today in the office.

The backdrop:

Around Thanksgiving last year, Dr. Aldrich snuck into the ofice and scared the living poop out of Annie, a cleaner and caretaker of the office. Turnabout is fair play.... See More

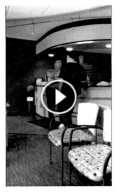

Like   Comment   Share   👍 26   💬 1   ↗ 1

 The Family Dental Center added 4 new photos to the album: April Fool's Day.
April 1, 2013

This is how we celebrate April Fool's at The Family Dental Center. It's all out of love:)

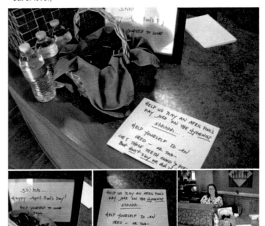

Like   Comment   Share   👍 34   💬 1

34.   Raffles & Guessing Games

Raffles and guessing games are like the lottery. Many will play, few will win. But they're always fun. You can create a number of fun raffles for your patients with various prizes. For example, anyone that "likes" a particular photo you post on Facebook can be entered in a drawing to win a gift certificate to the mall or a pair of movie tickets. Or have fun giveaways from a raffle of the month's "No Cavity Club".

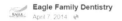
Eagle Family Dentistry
April 7, 2014

What's better than a free $50 gift card to The Garden Mart??? How about TWO free gift cards!

We're doubling down on our giveaway--1) LIKE this page and 2) SHARE this post by Wednesday for a chance to win! Your odds just got twice as good!

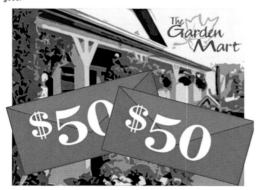

Like Comment Share 👍 48 💬 4 ↪ 62

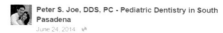
Peter S. Joe, DDS, PC - Pediatric Dentistry in South Pasadena
June 24, 2014

After your appointment, patients can guess how many soccer balls are in this jar. Each week, the closest guess will win one of these World Cup prizes! Let the guessing begin!

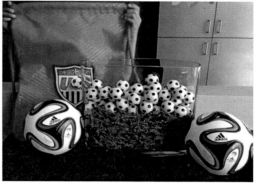

Like Comment Share 👍 6 💬 1

A guessing game can be set up at the front desk with a number of items, for example candy or even Cerec Blocs, into a jar. Have patients submit their best guess for how many are in the jar after their appointments. Post the jar on Facebook to let everyone know about the game, where they can submit their guesses via the comments section too. Have a gift handy for the winner and a photo opportunity with the winner as another Facebook post.

35.   No Cavities & Perfect Check-ups

Does your office do anything special for patients with good check-ups? Many offices feature a "No Cavity Club" for kids or a "Smile of the Month" for adults. For example, have a running list of all the kids during a given month that present with no cavities. Enter their names in a jar for a monthly drawing.

You can either take their picture at each "perfect check-up" to be entered into the drawing or have them swing by the office for a picture to receive their gift. A similar setup can be done for adults.

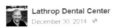

Lathrop Dental Center
December 30, 2014

Congrats Jacque and Coltyn! No cavities!!!

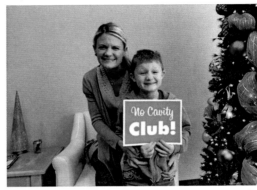

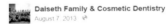
Like Comment Share 👍 24 💬 3

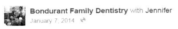

Bondurant Family Dentistry with Jennifer
January 7, 2014

Looking Pretty!

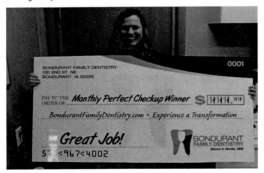

Like Comment Share 👍 26 💬 5

Dalseth Family & Cosmetic Dentistry
August 7, 2013

And the winners for July Cavity Free Club are: Ryder, Ava, and Emma. I know one girls who looks pretty psyched to be a winner of a Target gift card. Congratulations!

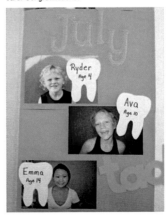

Like Comment Share 👍 9 💬 1

36. Dentists at the Dentist

For whatever reason, it's rather fascinating to patients when dentists get cavities. I believe the popularity of these types of posts, beyond the irony, is that you are portraying trust and confidence in your employees. Whether it's a filling or a cleaning, the fact that co-workers in the office have their dental work done by each other displays a favorable and marketable environment. Plus – it's fun(ny)!

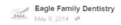

Eagle Family Dentistry
May 9, 2014

Even dentists need to go to the dentist!

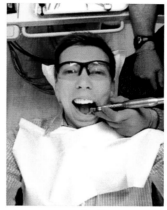

Like Comment Share 👍 22 💬 5

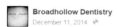

Broadhollow Dentistry
December 11, 2014

Dr. Chris gets a filling from a pregnant Dr. Erin and a pregnant Maria. We'll miss them when they're on maternity leave!

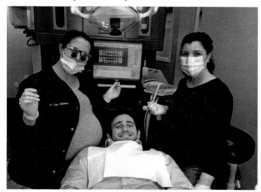

Like Comment Share 👍 70 💬 11

Bondurant Family Dentistry
August 12, 2013

Brayten showing Dr. Neville how it should be done!

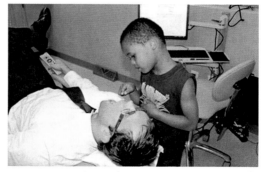

Like Comment Share 👍 93 💬 4 ↪ 1

37.   Little Helpers

Have any of your patients come to their cleaning appointment with their son or daughter? Kids are pretty darn cute, but they can be a bit nosy too. Sometimes they want to see what you're doing or to get in on the action themselves. So let them! Give them a mask and get a picture of the dentist-in-the-making!

 Great Florida Smiles & Orthodontics at **Great Florida Smiles & Orthodontics**
February 6

Better than any intern - the sweet little voice of Megan (Dr. Mike's daughter) asking, 'Can I help?' 😊 She helped fold the T-shirts for our orthodontic gift bags - reason enough to be a patient here 😊

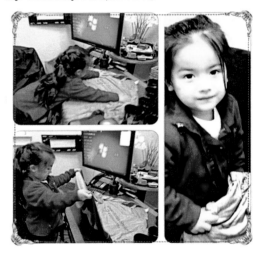

Like   Comment   Share   👍 23

 Wenatchee Pediatric Dentistry with Amber   and Christy
March 4 2014 Edited

What good helpers! Abby and sister, Peyton are assisting Amber with Parker's visit. Too much fun going on over here!! Happy Tuesday everyone!

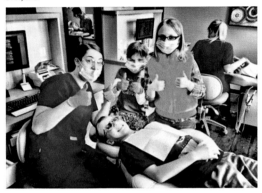

Like   Comment   Share   👍 60 💬 9

 Abbadent Family & Cosmetic Dentistry
November 8, 2014 Edited

I started Fastbraces on my wife Shelli recently and had one of the best assistants I could ask for! My daughter Landry was a great helper! Dr. Rauen

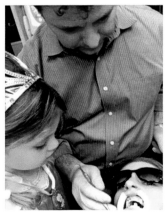

Unlike   Comment   Share   👍 48 💬 4 ↪ 1

38.　Braces Off

If your practice provides orthodontic treatment, the day that a patient gets his or her braces off is a big deal! Many orthodontists use this as a photo opportunity to take a picture of the patient and a staff member as a post in a weekly or monthly album. Alternatively you can also post before/after pictures of the big difference you've made. As always, you'll get the parent's release for photos of minors as well.

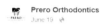
Prero Orthodontics
June 19

Congratulations Raquel on your beautiful new smile! It was a privilege to treat you 😊

We wish you the best of luck next year in college on the east coast. Your bright smile will take the California sun with you☺

Your Mom, and all of us at Prero Orthodontics are so proud of all of your accomplishments!... See More

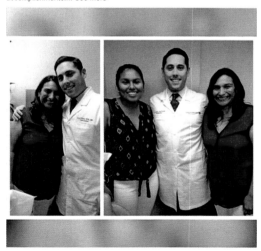

Like　Comment　Share　👍 15　↪ 1

Gorczyca Orthodontics - Antioch, CA
August 4, 2014

No more braces! Cameron enjoys soccer, cycling, and dirt bikes. We at Gorczyca Orthodontics think "You're the best!"

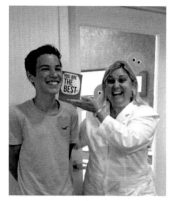

Like　Comment　Share　👍 5

Abbadent Family & Cosmetic Dentistry
March 15, 2013

So excited for Lisa and her awesome smile. She completed Fastbraces in less than 12 months!

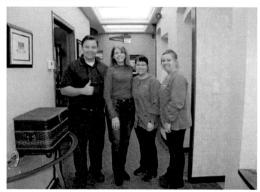

Like　Comment　Share　👍 5

39.   Shark Week

Chances are someone in your office gets all geeked-up about Shark Week. Shark Week is an annual, week-long block on the Discovery Channel that features shark-related programming. And it's a big deal, whether you know it or not. In fact it's hard to watch TV or even log into Facebook without seeing shark references or shark-based advertising during Shark Week. The media has a frenzy with Shark Week, so there's always shareable content floating around from magnificent pictures to comics and fun facts. For example, did you know that sharks can't get cavities? It's true - their teeth are coated with fluoride!

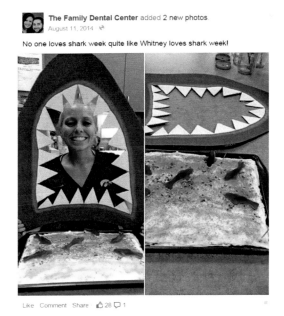

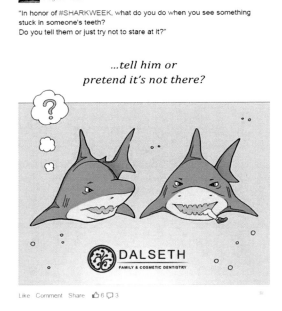

40. Olympics, Super Bowl & Major Sporting Events

The Olympic Games don't come around too often, but they sure are a world-wide sensation when they do! If you have televisions in your office, you can play the games on them so fans won't miss a beat. You should also be cheering for your favorite sports, events, countries or athletes on Facebook.

Hockey, soccer, football and other sports also usually have other news stories that accompany them, so feel free to comment on the headlines or share articles about the occasional athlete that breaks a tooth.

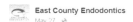

East County Endodontics
May 27

Go Warriors!!! Team Endo showing support for tonights game!

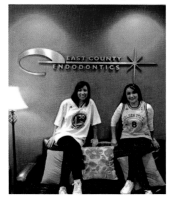

Like   Comment   Share   👍15 💬1

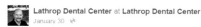

Lathrop Dental Center at Lathrop Dental Center
January 30

2 Seahawks Vs. 5 Patriots...
Who is your Super Bowl pick?

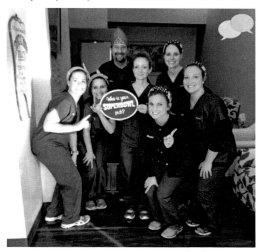

Like   Comment   Share   👍19 💬8 ↪1

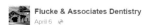

Flucke & Associates Dentistry
April 6

We are supporting our boys in blue for opening day!

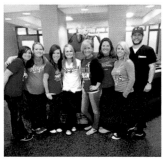

Like   Comment   Share   👍24 💬3

41. Sports Rivalries

Got a favorite sports team? Any rivalries in the office? Set up a March Madness bracket within the office. Maybe one of the dentists went to a neighboring state's dental school and the two are playing each other on Saturday. Wear your colors, get a bobble-head mascot on the front desk, hang up some flags or posters. Just keep it positive, and don't get into any bitter arguments in the comments section!

 Marshalltown Family Dentistry
September 11 at 8:39am

An office divided! But we are ALL looking forward to the game:) Who will you be cheering for tomorrow?

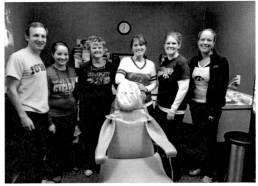

Like   Comment   Share   👍 33   💬 4

 Waterloo Dental Associates with Christopher Aldrich and Jill
August 28, 2014

Definitely some trash talk going on at WDA today!! Enjoy some football this weekend!

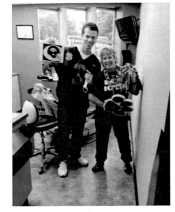

Like   Comment   Share   👍 47   💬 11

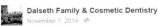 **Dalseth Family & Cosmetic Dentistry**
November 7, 2014

The border battle begins....who do you want to win Floyd of Rosedale?

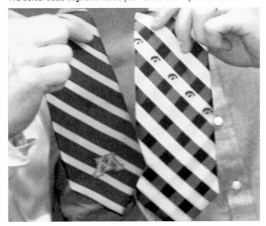

Like   Comment   Share   👍 4   💬 3   ↪ 1

42.   Local Events

Your attendance and participation at local events are a good way to integrate and interact with your community. Share a photo from the State Fair. Congratulate the team of local high school students that won the regional soccer game or science competition. Get involved!

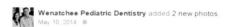

Wenatchee Pediatric Dentistry added 2 new photos.
May 10, 2014

Touch A Truck going strong!! What a great community event!

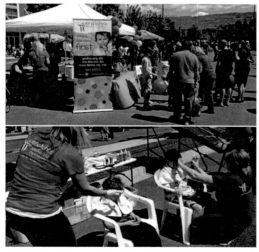

Like   Comment   Share   👍 24

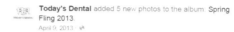

Today's Dental added 5 new photos to the album: Spring Fling 2013.
April 9, 2013

Did you attend Spring Fling 2013?! Take a look at some of the photos we took this year!

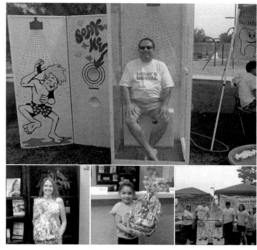

Like   Comment   Share   👍 5

43.   Local News

Are you known as the local expert in all things teeth and oral health related? You should be! Seek out and take advantage of every opportunity to be in the public eye (or ear if we're talking radio). Speak for the local nightly news. Become the go-to dentist with your local radio station. Sponsor a sports team or a float in the parade. There are many ways to cultivate these golden opportunities for great marketing.

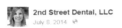

2nd Street Dental, LLC
July 8, 2014

Watch for Dr. Miranda's interview today on K2 News!

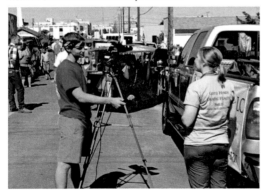

Like   Comment   Share   👍 31   ↪ 2

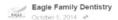

Eagle Family Dentistry
October 5, 2014

Here is Dr. Dulde's full interview with Trinity Broadcasting Network as a spokesperson for WDA's Own Your Smile campaign.

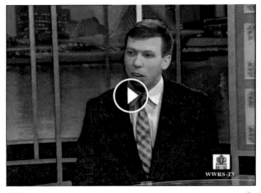

676 Views

Like   Comment   Share   👍 15   💬 3   ↪ 3

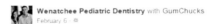

Wenatchee Pediatric Dentistry with GumChucks
February 6

Did you hear Dr. Ping on the air with Connor and Mel today? #kw3 #flosslikeaboss #brushtwiceflossonce

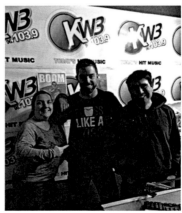

Like   Comment   Share   👍 37   💬 3

44.   Tooth Talks

Wondering how to build a reputation as the local tooth expert? Start small. Literally. Check with your local day care or elementary school to see if they could use a refresher on brushing and flossing. Have some fun facts, props and a few tricks up your sleeve. You may not inspire every child to brush twice a day, but the staff at the school, the parents and your patients will all praise and thank you for your efforts.

Eagle Family Dentistry added 5 new photos.
March 31, 2014

Thank you to LOVE, LAUGH, and LEARN for having us last Friday! We enjoyed spending the morning with all of your smiling faces!

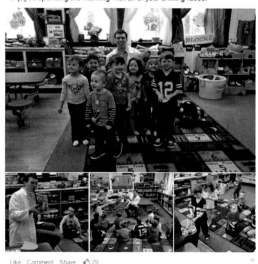

Like   Comment   Share   👍 29

Pediatric Dentistry with Jason Gonzalez
November 12, 2013

You might have heard... Dr. Gonzalez, our resident MAGICIAN has performed over 25 "oral health" magic shows in the Cheyenne/Laramie areas. The shows have been a hit with local day cares. If you know of a day care or group of young ones that would like to see the magic show, give us a call!

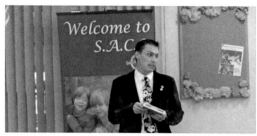

Unlike   Comment   Share   👍 204 💬 15 ↪ 11

Bondurant Family Dentistry added 4 new photos to the album: Tooth Talk — with Steven Neville and Joe
February 18, 2014

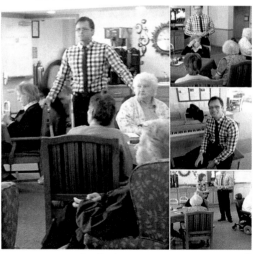

Like   Comment   Share   👍 97 💬 7 ↪ 1

Alternatively, a retirement community home is another great audience for a "tooth talk" or oral hygiene discussion.

45.   Bridal Shows, Expos and Exhibitions

What does every major dental CE meeting have in common? Exhibitor fairs! Look into your local community and I'll bet you find wedding expos, new mom's fairs and other events along those lines. These shows provide a great marketing opportunity whether the dentist attends or sends sociable staff members to represent the office.

Free whitening for the bride and groom? Perfect. Have some dental swag or a few gifts to raffle off? Even better. Set up a colorful booth and dress the part or wear team t-shirts!

 1st Family Dental at 1st Family Dental Of Fox Valley
July 17

Please join us in congratulating Jennifer & Tristan - the winners of our Wedding Whitening grand prize! This lovely couple is tying the knot in just 4 weeks, and after a visit to our office, they have smiles as bright as their future together. ♡

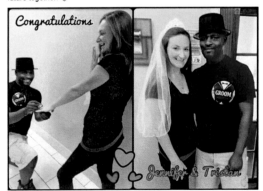

Like   Comment   Share   👍 84 💬 2 ↩ 3

 Watertown Dental Care with Ashley Pfrimmer
January 25 Edited

Visit our booth at the Prom and Bridal Showcase today in the Codington County Extension Complex! Dr. Ashley is presenting great information and fabulous offers on Six Month Smiles, Botox, Juvederm, & KoR Professional Whitening!

Watertown Dental Care is pleased to offer services to help you look and feel your best on your memorable day!

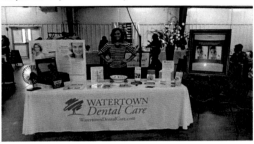

Like   Comment   Share   👍 16 💬 1

 The Family Dental Center shared their album
June 23, 2014

Check out photos from the Baby Talk Event! We had a blast!

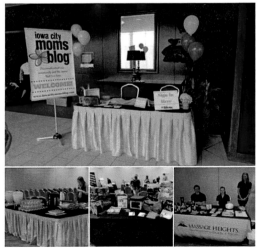

Like   Comment   Share   👍 7

46.   Vacations

Who doesn't love a good vacation? For example, if someone in the office recently got married, have them send back some of their best photos from the honeymoon. Share a photo or small collage and congratulate them. Any unique destination photos from any staff member can be shared.

The Family Dental Center added 5 new photos.
September 17, 2014

Katie is on vacation in Colorado & has been sending us pictures that look like they're right out of a nature magazine! Amazing!

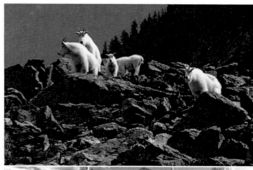

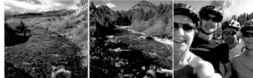

Like   Comment   Share   👍 29

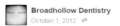

Broadhollow Dentistry
October 1, 2012

Maria got married yesterday! We'll miss her while she travels across Italy on her honeymoon!

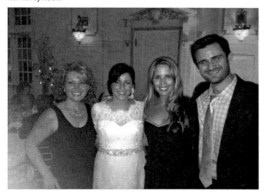

Like   Comment   Share   👍 14   💬 2

When done tastefully, i.e. without showing off that you are in Hawaii in the middle of February while everyone else is freezing their butts off, it can make for a fun and interesting post.

Dr. Michael Hopkins Dental Office at Ruby Mountain Heli Ski
February 9

Doc Hopkins powder skiing

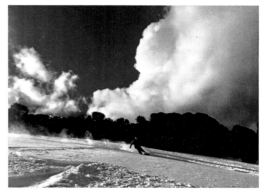

Like   Comment   Share   👍 68   💬 3

47. Historic Birthdays

In addition to the federal holidays commemorating historic birthdays, such as President's day or Martin Luther King, Jr day, other birthdays may deserve an honorable mention. Who in history inspires you? Look up their birthday and celebrate it on social media. For example, are you an Elvis fan? Dr. Seuss? Abe Lincoln? Most greats in history have inspirational quotes that they are known for. You can either find a photo and overlay your favorite quote with a photo editing app or search for one on Google. Here are some examples from the ones I mentioned.

"Ambition is a dream with a V8 engine." *–Elvis Presley*

"Why fit in? When you were born to stand out!" *–Dr. Seuss*

"Whatever you are, be a good one." *–Abraham Lincoln*

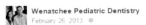

Wenatchee Pediatric Dentistry
February 26, 2013

"It all began with that shoe on the wall. A shoe on a wall...? Shouldn't be there at all!"

Are you celebrating Dr. Suess's birthday this week? It's a fun way to come up with activities for your children. May we suggest a Wacky Wednesday for your children? It can be as simple as putting things where they are not supposed to be and letting your children do a scavenger hunt to find all of the wacky, out of place things!

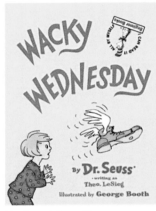

Like Comment Share 👍 8

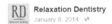

Relaxation Dentistry
January 8, 2014

Happy birthday Elvis from all of us at Relaxation Dentistry!

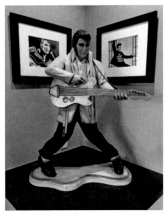

Like Comment Share 👍 7

48.   Dental Holidays

Believe it or not, there are several holidays for the dental profession. They usually don't receive national recognition but they can and should be celebrated within the dental community and certainly within your dental office.

First is National Dentist's Day on March 6th of each year. This day is all about the dentists in the office. A group photo of the docs is a must.

Dental Assistant Appreciation Week also happens to be the first full week of March. Do something special for the assistants. Either feature each of them throughout the week or have flowers or a cake ready for them, thanking them for all they do.

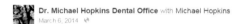

Dr. Michael Hopkins Dental Office with Michael Hopkins
March 6, 2014

Happy National Dentist's Day to two of the best dentists we know! Thank you for taking such great pride in the work you do and being such great bosses as well! #NationalDentistDay

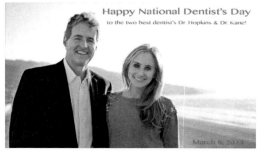

Like   Comment   Share   👍 16 💬 1

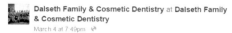

Dalseth Family & Cosmetic Dentistry at Dalseth Family & Cosmetic Dentistry
March 4 at 7:49pm

This week is Assistant Appreciation Week. When you are in, make sure to tell them what a great job they do!

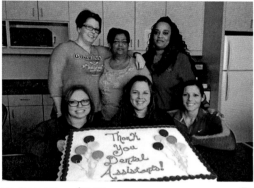

Like   Comment   Share   👍 24 💬 1

National Dental Hygienists week is the second week of April. This is their week, not to be confused with National Dental Hygiene month which is October.

And for the front office, there's also an Administration Day that is observed on the last Wednesday of April. A list of all relevant dates are listed in the next chapter.

49.   Office Construction

Who likes dealing with construction? I certainly don't. But it's a necessary evil. Turn it into a positive and send out a "sorry for the inconvenience" but also let everyone know how helpful this project will be in treating your patients. Even smaller projects like a new bulletin board for the "No Cavity Club" or a new piece of dental equipment deserves a post. Remember to focus on the features and benefits for your patients.

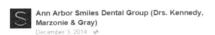

Ann Arbor Smiles Dental Group (Drs. Kennedy, Marzonie & Gray)
December 3, 2014

We're going green!

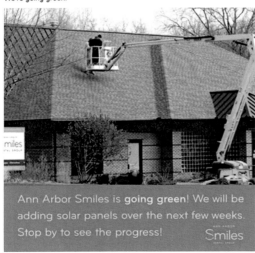

Unlike Comment Share 👍 12 💬 1

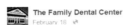

The Family Dental Center
February 18

The finishing touches. We're almost done with our new additions!

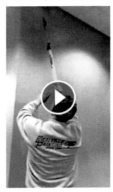

569 Views
Like Comment Share 👍 23 💬 3

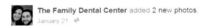

The Family Dental Center added 2 new photos.
January 21

I think the hard hats are a nice touch. Safety first! 😊

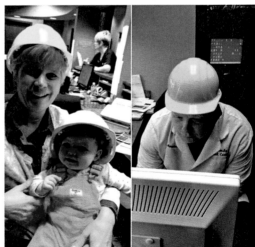

Like Comment Share 👍 45 💬 3 ↗ 1

50.   Last Days & Retirement

Whether it's your retirement or that of a staff member, or even someone moving or taking on a new job, it can and should be celebrated. Snap a couple photos at the retirement party, with their flowers or gifts and provide a thoughtful caption. Some prefer a calm, quiet getaway while others will throw confetti and go dancing down the hallways. Either way, retirement is a big deal! Reflect on their fruitful career and the impact they've made. Don't let it go unnoticed!

 Waterloo Dental Associates with Marsha
August 7, 2014

Congratulations to Marsha on her last day today before retirement!! She has been an amazing part of WDA for 28 years! She will be greatly missed!!!

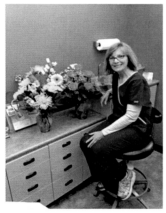

Like Comment Share   👍 70 💬 26 ↪ 1

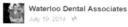 **Waterloo Dental Associates**
July 19, 2014

"The retirement dance!"

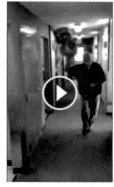

Unlike Comment Share   👍 65 💬 12 ↪ 1

The Family Dental Center added 2 new photos
September 18 at 9:00am

Today is Whitney's last day with us at The Family Dental Center. Good luck in your new adventures! We will miss you!

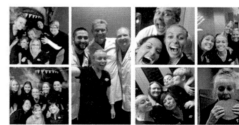

Like Comment Share   👍 28 💬 2

6 HOLIDAYS AND IMPORTANT DATES

Y ou probably keep a personal calendar in your home or office. It's a great way to mark important dates, such as the birthdays of your family and friends. This calendar may cue you to call or text these people on those special days. Or maybe you rely solely on the Facebook notification to write them a quick message on their wall. A similar calendar of holidays and events can be kept for your social media efforts. It should include all major holidays, from federal to unofficial or local dates that you can post on. It should also include the birthdays of each and every staff member, as well as work anniversaries for each employee. You can also include the date when your practice opened its doors to reflect humbly on your career, the satisfaction your patients bring you and the history of the practice every year.

Once a month or so, perhaps during your team meetings, review the upcoming dates and events. Also mention the plan or brainstorm how to commemorate each important date in the office and/or on Facebook. And of course, have your cameras (phones) ready to capture the Kodak moments. It may be tough to remember at first, but once the social culture is implemented, it'll become second nature to document these memories and share them with your audience.

Below is a list of post-worthy dates that you can transfer to the social calendar for your practice. Some dates may vary from year to year. Google any questionable dates to confirm their accuracy.

January

Near Year's Day	Jan 1
Martin Luther King Jr Day	Third Monday of Jan

February

National Children's Dental Health Month	
Black History Month	
Groundhog Day	Feb 2
National Wear Red Day	First Friday of February
Abraham Lincoln's Birthday	Feb 12
Valentine's Day	Feb 14
President's Day	Third Monday of Feb
National Tooth Fairy Day	February 28 (some sources say August 22)

March

Women's History Month	
Dental Assistant Appreciation Week	First full week of March
Dr. Seuss's Birthday	March 2
National Dentist's Day	March 6
Pi Day	March 14
Saint Patrick's Day	March 17
National Puppy Day	March 23
Daylight Saving Time (US)	Varies annually
First Day of Spring	Varies annually
Root Canal Awareness Week	Varies annually

April

Oral Cancer Awareness Month	
Prosthodontics Awareness Week	Varies annually
National Dental Hygienists Week	Second week of April
April Fool's Day	April 1
National Volunteer Week	Varies annually
Good Friday	Friday before Easter
Easter	Various Sundays
National Siblings Day	April 10
Earth Day	April 22
DNA Day	April 25
Administrative Professionals Day	Last Wednesday of April
Arbor Day	Last Friday of April

May

National Pet Month	
Star Wars Day	May 4
Mother's Day	Second Sunday of May
Memorial Day	Last Monday of May

June

Flag Day	June 14
Father's Day	Third Sunday of June
First Day of Summer	Varies annually
National Toothbrush Day	June 26

July

Independence Day	July 4
Ice Cream Day	Third Sunday in July

August

Shark Week	Varies annually
National Tooth Fairy Day	August 22 (some sources say February 28)

September

Labor Day	First Monday of Sep
Patriot Day	Sep 11
First Day of Fall	Varies annually

October

National Dental Hygiene Month	
Boss's Day	October 16
Columbus Day	Second Monday of Oct
Mole Day	Oct 23
Halloween	Oct 31
Day of the Dead (Mexico)	Oct 31

November

American Diabetes Month	
No-Shave November (Movember)	
Election day	Tues following First Mon
Daylight Saving Time (US)	Varies annually
Veterans Day	Usually Nov 11

Thanksgiving	Fourth Thursday of Nov
Black Friday	Friday after Thanksgiving
Small Business Saturday	Saturday after Thanksgiving
Cyber Monday	Monday after Thanksgiving

December

Pearl Harbor Day	Dec 7
First Day of Winter	Varies annually
Festivus	Dec 23
Christmas	Dec 25

Customize your social calendar as you see fit. Pick your favorite holidays and make it a celebration. Have a few favorite hobbies? Do a search to see if there are any special or commemorative dates that celebrate these events or activities. Share your involvement or appreciation on these days.

"Keep a social calendar."

7 FACEBOOK INSIGHTS

Measuring success on social media is about more than counting your likes. Insights is a free analysis tool that allows you to learn more about your Facebook audience and their interactions with your page. Found above your cover photo within the administrator tabs, Insights consists of six subcategories: Overview, Likes, Reach, Visits, Posts and People. This chapter reviews the key components of each.

Page   Messages   Notifications   **Insights**   Posts   Export   Settings   Help ·

OVERVIEW

The "Overview" tab gives you a snapshot of your stats [Likes, Reach, Engagement] for this week compared to last week. Depending on how often you post, this may or may not be very useful. Let's face it, some content is more interesting than other content, and consequently some weeks are better than others. Of course the goal is to achieve a general increase in fans and engagement, but don't beat yourself up if you have a down week here and there. Furthermore it may be difficult to read the line graphs without correlating the highs and the lows with specific posts, which is why I find the next section more useful.

"Your 5 Most Recent Posts" (next page). The most intuitive and useful information from this category are the Reach and Engagement columns. They provide a great visual snapshot of the performance of your recent posts in a color coordinated display.

Published ▼	Post	Type	Targeting	Reach		Engagement		Promote
03/19/2015 9:34 pm	So apparently not everyone thinks typodonts are awesome?!?	🔗	🌐	36K		3.9K 856		Boost Post
03/18/2015 8:31 am	DENTISTS: Have you experienced this today? #StPatricks #DayAfter #EmergencyVisits	🔗	🌐	3.3K		126 12		Boost Post
03/17/2015 4:54 pm	Happy St Paddy's Day and remember to floss!!!	🗐	🌐	11.4K		171 623		Boost Post
03/13/2015 10:17 am	Does it get any nerdier than this? Happy Friday the 13th! #dentalhumor #tooth13	🗐	🌐	61.8K		935 3K		Boost Post
03/11/2015 8:10 am	"Louis! Let's do this!" -Stewie Start the brushing routine early with your child to help make it a habit.	🗐	🌐	1.8K		92 34		Boost Post

Scrolling past your recent posts brings you to "Pages to Watch". Facebook suggests 5 "similar" Facebook pages and allows you to compare some of your statistics to the pages you select, allowing you to compare total page likes, new page likes, number of posts this week and their engagement for the week. You can select from the pages that Facebook suggests, or you can find various pages that you are either interested in keeping up with or dental pages that you admire for comparison. You can also start a friendly competition with practice pages of your dental friends from surrounding areas.

LIKES

The "Likes" tab provides the numbers for your Facebooks fans over time and where they came from. A slender graph at the top provides an overview of the past three months and below that we find a slightly more detailed diagram of your Total Page Likes.

Next are your "Net Likes" which balance your number of new likes with your unlikes. Most people that like a business page do not unlike that page, unless the page violates some of the rules we have set forth, i.e. overbearing self-promotions, calls to action with no value, posting too frequently or not frequently enough, etc.

"Where Your Page Likes Happened" gives a breakdown of how your fans found your page. The categories are vague, and I've found that most fans come from your page, from a mysterious "uncategorized mobile" source or from a search.

REACH

The "Reach" tab is another indicator of your performance over time. While I think reach is very valuable, the way it is represented in this tab is with a line graph, which I find difficult to interpret or correlate with specific posts, so the utility of this tab may be somewhat limited.

Post Reach

The number of people your post was served to.

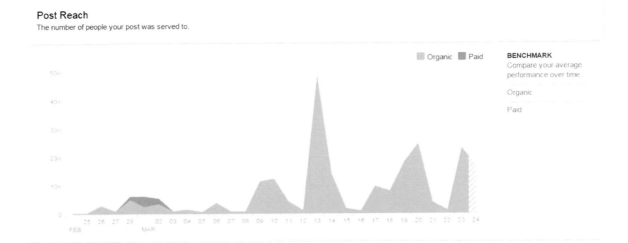

"Post Reach" (pictured) reveals how many people saw your posts over the past month. Post Reach is one of the most important metrics for you page as it conveys each post's relative success. This category also segregates your organic from your paid reach. For example, if you boosted a post, you will see a representation of the difference boosting made for that post.

"Likes, Comments and Shares" are the engagements that your posts received over time. In general, you will get more likes than comments and more comments than shares.

Hopefully you don't have too many "Hide, Report as Spam and Unlikes". These actions will tend to decrease your reach. As mentioned, most people won't hide or unlike your page unless you annoy or offend them. Also, as patients move or otherwise leave the practice, they may unlike your page as it becomes irrelevant for them.

"Total Reach" is a graphical overview of your comprehensive reach over time.

VISITS

"Page and Tab Visits" reveals where people spent their time on your page between your timeline, photos tab, likes tab, info tab or any other tabs that you created for your page.

"External references" reviews how some of your fans came across your Facebook page.

POSTS

The "Posts" tab is divided into three subcategories: When your fans are online, Post Types and Top Posts from Pages to Watch.

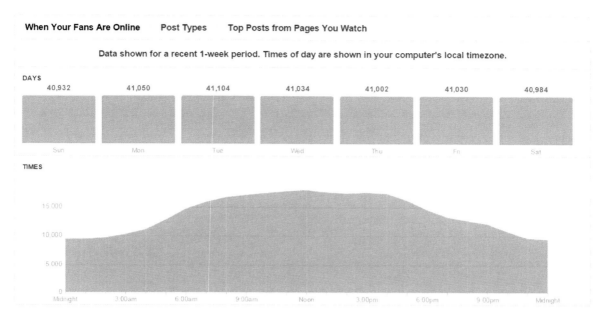

"When Your Fans Are Online" (pictured). Scroll through the days of the week and assess when most of your fans are online. Across Facebook, this usually occurs along a bell-shaped curve that ascends in the morning, peaks around noon time and starts to descend again during the early evening hours. Check the specifics for your Facebook fans because "when your fans are online" actually translates to *when you should post your Facebook posts*. Post sometime during the ascent, or if your online times plateau for several hours, schedule your posts to deploy within the first half of the plateau. Facebook gives most posts about 5 hours to reach their audience and allow fans to engage with the content. If no engagement occurs, the post diminishes from timelines and fades from view. Engagements, including clicks, likes, comments, etc. prolong the

life of a post and the post can recirculate into your fans' timelines for hours, sometimes days, after its debut.

"Post types" compares the success of various types of posts including status updates, links and photos based on reach, post clicks and other engagements (likes, comments, shares).

If you are keeping track of other pages, "Top Posts from Pages You Watch" will let your compare your posts to some of their recent posts.

At the bottom of each subcategory within the Posts tab, you'll see "All Posts Published". This provides the same information as "Your 5 Most Recent Posts" from the Overview tab, but also allows you to browse through all of your posts. Once every few months, take a

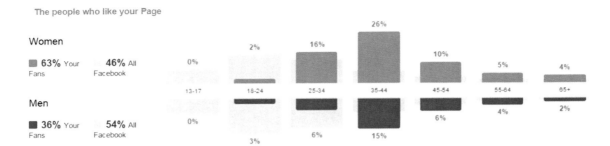

The people who like your Page

Women

■ **63%** Your Fans **46%** All Facebook

Men

■ **36%** Your Fans **54%** All Facebook

look back and assess your most successful posts. Analyze them to learn what set these posts apart. Was it a particular holiday? What time of day did you post? Was it geared toward a certain age group? Was it particularly personal? Did it evoke certain emotions? If you have several staff administrators that help co-manage and create content for your page, you can use this tab to see which staff member is putting out the most successful content. If you host a friendly monthly or quarterly "most social" competition, get them something nice for a job well done!

PEOPLE

The "People" tab is also divided into several categories: Your Fans, People Reached and People Engaged. This tab is easily one of the most useful analyses that Insights provides.

"Your Fans" (pictured) provides the demographic breakdown of your Facebook fans. At the top you'll find men, women and their respective age groups. In blue are your fans and in gray is Facebook at large. For general dentists, the composition of your fans

should, more or less, mirror the demographic of your patients. For pediatric and orthodontic practices, your fans may reflect the parents of your patients and may also be weighted with a younger audience if a portion of your pediatric patients like you on Facebook. However, your posts and marketing should be geared towards kid-friendly and parent-friendly content. Further down we see the numbers by country, city and language. The city category, of course, will prove most relevant in terms of your reach as a practitioner in the area.

The "People" tab can also be an important indicator for the authenticity of your fans. Some dental practices partner with marketers to manage their social media activity. If you've hired out that function and your Facebook following exploded overnight, check this tab in your Insights. Purchased "likes" usually sway your fan demographics and many appear from foreign countries. So if you practice in Walnut Creek, California and half of your fans are from India, you may have fallen into the trap. Although Facebook has recently tried to curtail fake and inactive accounts, phony

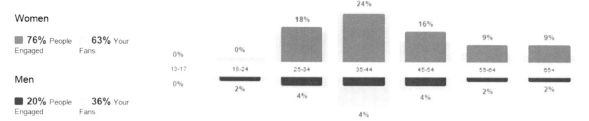

The people who have liked, commented on, or shared your posts or engaged with your Page in the past 28 days.

Women

■ **76%** People Engaged   **63%** Your Fans

Men

■ **20%** People Engaged   **36%** Your Fans

likes still plague some social media pages. The problem is that you may be broadcasting your content to a false viewer and these accounts do not engage with your content, so they won't improve your reach. To my knowledge, there is no way to individually delete these accounts from your Facebook fans. As with most things, prevention is best. One way to work around the situation is to target each of your posts to your city or state, though this can be cumbersome in its own right.

"People Reached" is another valuable tab that shows the breakdown of the population you are reaching with your posts. Analyze the makeup of your reach. Are you reaching the audience you intended? If you aren't, you may want to look a second look at your content. Is it appropriate for the demographic of the audience you are trying to reach?

Also keep in mind that certain groups of people, i.e. young women, tend to engage more on social media. You can view the subgroups of those that engaged with your content in the "People Engaged" tab (pictured).

> *"Measuring success is about more than counting likes."*

8 OTHER SOCIAL MEDIA PLATFORMS

B ased on the numbers, Facebook is still king of today's social media domain. But while it may be the biggest player, other social media platforms have not only made a name for themselves but hold precedence when it comes to select features, characteristics and niche markets. More social media platforms exist today than any one person can conquer and maintain. As is advised for most small businesses, picking 2 or 3 social media platforms that work best with your office and your patients is usually the most appropriate method. Joining some merely for the possibility of a small boost in search engine rankings is also fair game.

When choosing which outlets your practice will participate in, consider several factors. The most important of which is the demographic makeup of your patients and your target audience. These two are not necessarily the same. For example, pediatric and orthodontic practices may not aim to market and communicate directly with their young patients but rather their parents. Another consideration is the preferences of you and your staff. Some members of your staff may already be well versed in certain platforms. Is there an artist or photographer among your staff that loves taking and editing pictures? Instagram would be an easy addition to the repertoire. Someone at the front desk "pinning" in their free time? Add Pinterest to the list.

Some social media services allow you to sync one another. The most notable of which is synching Twitter to Facebook so that when you post to one, the other automatically posts the same content. However, beware that they don't share complete continuity. For example, even when you have them synched, posting a picture to Facebook shows up as a link on Twitter that leads back to the original Facebook post. A similar phenomenon results between Twitter and Instagram. This hardly makes for a great user experience, but these proprietary antics are imposed to make sure users are using *their* sites and posting content to *their* platforms.

One way to get around this is to use social media management services. These programs allow you to manage several social media accounts from a central hub or dashboard. For example, a service called Hootsuite allows you to schedule posts that appear in native form to Facebook, Twitter, Google+ and now Instagram. Hootsuite allows you to manage up to 3 social media accounts for free and enables abbreviated links. Give it a try.

You can also download supplementary photo and video editing apps to optimize your photographs or videos. Download and play around with a few, such as Quick, PicLab, Color Cap and others. See which one(s) you like best and pay the couple dollars it costs to edit your pictures without their logo on it and to unlock all of their features.

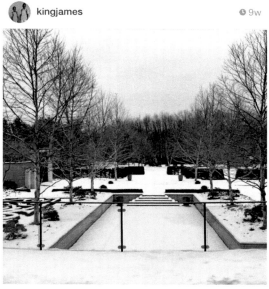

201,585 likes

kingjames I love it!!! Home Sweet Home

INSTAGRAM

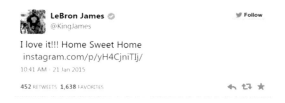

TWITTER

A review of the major social media outlets follows with quick facts, summaries of unique features and my opinion on their place in dentistry.

TWITTER

- Founded: March 2006
- Posts are called "tweets"
- Hashtags (#)
- User tags (@)
- Similar to Facebook now

- 284M active users (world)
- 50M active users (US)
- 2nd largest social media network
- Can be synched with Facebook

What made Twitter special in the early years was its simplicity. It was unique in that it allowed only 140 characters of text in each post – nothing more, nothing less. Everything that you wanted to express was to fit in that window with a message, a link, a hashtag (#) and/or tagging another user with the "@" symbol. For those of you that are still in the dark about hashtags, it is simply a way to tag your post with a keyword or phrase. It can also be used to add flare or ironic humor to a post. If it's a popular term that users are interested in, your content can be found amongst all of the other posts using this same hashtag.

Today, Twitter looks a lot like the Facebook timeline, allowing users to attach photos, videos and music to their tweets. Twitter is especially prominent in the news and entertainment industry, allowing users to interact with celebrities and television programming. One key difference lies in the stringent privacy settings of Facebook that many users utilize. Twitter, on the other hand, is more of an "open book" where user profiles are kept public. This can be useful for companies or brands interested in learning more about their customers.

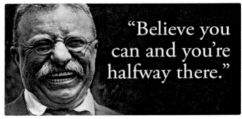

For your dental practice, I recommend having a Twitter account. Ideally, you would either post content directly through Twitter or a social media management service to assure a native or optimized display of content. Synching Twitter and Facebook is a "quick and dirty" trick, and content created on Facebook won't be optimized for Twitter. But if you're not willing to give Twitter its own special time, it may at least be worth synching to show face on another platform and add the little bird to the social media bar on your website.

GOOGLE+

- Founded: June 2011
- Similar to Facebook
- Register website

- 300+M users (sort of)
- Estimated 35% users active
- SEO boost

Google muscled its way into the social media stratosphere in 2011. It was slow to start and met some resistance, but has maintained itself mainly as a means for users to access Gmail, YouTube and other Google services, and for businesses to optimize their ranking within Google's search engine. Your website must be registered with Google in order to be found on search, Maps and Google+. Your website developer has likely completed this task for you, otherwise it is free to do so yourself.

Content is similar to Facebook in that it includes pictures, videos, links and tags, but differs slightly in format to include 2-3 columns of content. You won't gather a substantial patient following on Google+. Similar to your Blog, staying active on Google+ may benefit your SEO ranking within Google searches. This is a hassle, but can be conveniently added to your collection when using a social media management service such as Hootsuite.

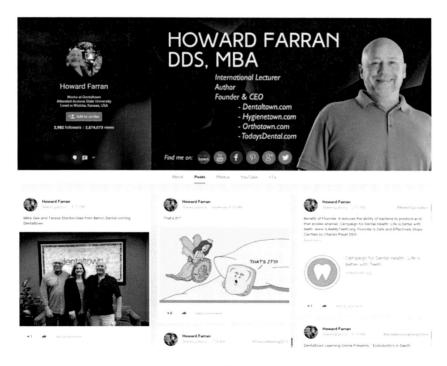

LinkedIn

- Founded: December 2002
- News feed similar to Facebook
- SEO boost
- 300+M users
- Create a business page

LinkedIn is known as the "professional" social network. Content from your friends and selected businesses show up on your News Feed in a similar fashion to Facebook. For the personal user, a profile is created that is similar to a resume or C.V. In fact many businesses use LinkedIn as a means for recruitment, and users can endorse each other for various skills and expertise.

I recommend creating a personal profile as well as a Company Page for your practice. While you may be able to form connections between your personal friends as well as others in the dental field, you will not build a large network from within your patients. Your profile and practice page may add a small benefit to SEO, but don't spend too much time getting fancy with LinkedIn.

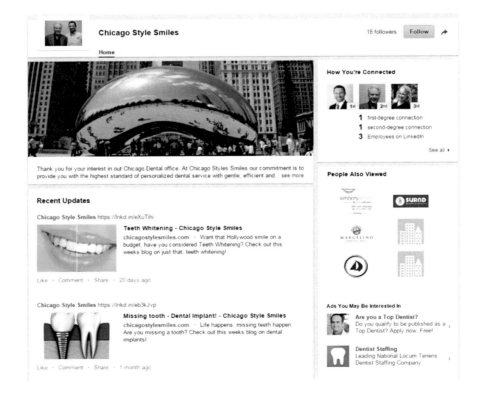

INSTAGRAM

- Founded: October 2010
- Owned by Facebook
- Hashtags (#) and user tags (@)
- Edit your photographs
- 300+M active users (world)
- 45+M active users (US)
- Does not allow links in individual posts

In April of 2012, Facebook acquired Instagram for $1 billion, a bargain considering Instagram's tremendous growth and popularity. Not to mention Facebook's subsequent purchase of a messaging app for $19 billion just two years later. Instagram is an app that allows users to enhance their photographs and short videos by adding a variety of filters and other enhancements to the visuals. Instagram continues to grow with the largest group of users between 16-24 years of age followed by 25-34 year olds.

Due to the inherent settings of the app, it has limited potential for a dental practice in terms of growing an audience. While Instagram allows links in a user's bio or front page, it does not allow links to be placed in individual posts. Instagram is also not as public a platform as the others. You receive notifications when other users like or comment on your content, but that won't show up on any of their friend's content feeds. I have, however, personally seen some dental practices using the platform effectively and successfully, especially pediatric and orthodontic practices.

If you are new to Instagram, download the app and play around with it. You may find that you like to edit or enhance some photographs before you post them to other platforms. If you take enough photographs or video and the motivation to stay active on Instagram, it may be an effective platform for you. If you or your staff do not use it consistently, I wouldn't bother asking patients to follow you on Instagram.

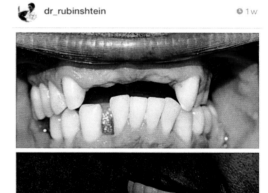

143 likes

dr_rubinshtein Before: Patient "I'm tired of not smiling" After: Patient "My face hurts from smiling" 😊😊😊😊😊 #tuesday #transformation #smile #makeover #dentist #nyc #miami #cosmeticdentistry #details #stpatricksday #alldent

view all 11 comments

PINTEREST

- Founded: March 2010
- 65% users 16-34 years old
- 70M users
- Up to 80% women

Pinterest is yet another visually inclined platform, allowing users to create pin-up board style pages with anything that interests them. The majority of users on Pinterest are young females between the ages of 16-34 years. As such, the most popular categories on Pinterest are food, drink and crafts, rightfully termed "Pinterest projects".

Interestingly, images without faces are 23% more likely to be re-pinned. This suggests that, unlike Facebook, Pinterest is more about things than people. If you or any of your staff are well versed on Pinterest and your target audience is the young female population, Pinterest may be a good fit for your practice.

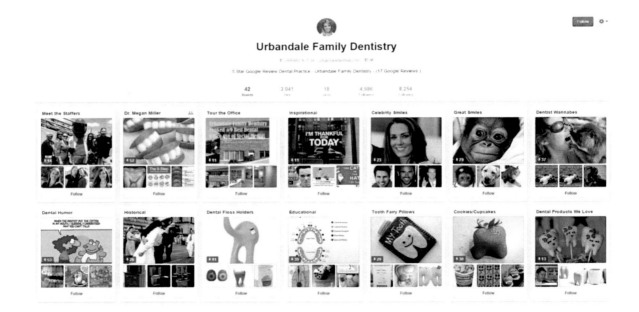

SNAPCHAT

- Founded: September 2011
- Most users are young
- Unknown metrics
- Limited use for dental

Snapchat is one of the hottest new tickets in social media. Facebook was turned down for their offer to buy Snapchat in 2013 for $3 billion in cash. The premise of Snapchat is to send short picture or video messages, with captions or on-screen drawings, that disappear once viewed. Snapchat has added various features such as text messages and Stories that can be shared and allow your friends to see your content for up to 24 hours. It is a growing platform, particularly with teenagers and young adults, though Snapchat keeps a tight lid on its exact metrics and user data.

Some companies are experimenting with Snapchat to reach consumers. In its current state, it presents limited uses for the average dental practice. I can conjure a scenario where a pediatric or orthodontic practice may distribute comical or entertaining visual messages related to oral hygiene to a younger audience, but I am not aware of any dental practices that have incorporated Snapchat into their lineup yet. If you or any of your dental acquaintances are using Snapchat, I would love to hear from you!

VINE

- Founded: January 2013
- Owned by Twitter
- 40M users
- Limited use for dental

Like Snapchat, Vine is one of the newer social networks with a growing, but youthful audience, particularly in the 13-24 year range. Vine is a video sharing service that sets a 7-second timer for its video bits.

Vine is also similar to Snapchat in that I do not know any dental practices that utilize Vine for marketing purposes.

"Pick 2 or 3 that work best for your practice."

9 FINAL THOUGHTS

As you may have noticed – technology is moving fast and getting faster. We live in a time where we reach to our phones for restaurant recommendations on the weekends. We hail a cab with the click of a button instead of a wave of the hand or even a phone call. We swipe left or right to find love on dating apps and we push a button on our laundry machine for delivery service when we are running low on detergent. Times have certainly changed. Technology has driven this change and digitalized many aspects of our lives.

Marketing is no exception. Throughout history, marketing efforts have focused on the mediums with the most prominent and active audiences. And each new form of media has tended to leach the masses from its predecessor. Radio from print, television from radio and the internet from all three sources. Social media, an evolutionary branch of the internet, is on course to shift the paradigm yet again for all media sources. And it is doing so at record speeds. Thirty-eight years passed before 50 million people had access to radios. Television grew to that size in just thirteen years. Instagram? Eighteen months. Social media is no longer the new kid on the block. It is an established and influential marketing platform that is making the world a little smaller, more transparent and more connected every day.

My goal in writing this book was to help good dentists effectively deliver their message through social media to an ever more savvy and informed audience. We know the numbers when it comes to social media – and they are staggering. Social media is so ubiquitous that it simply cannot be ignored. Literally! Take a look around. Out on a busy street. In line at the grocery store. At the gym between sets. People are on their phones *a lot*. And if you want to get your message across, that's where you should be too.

Gone are the days of the Yellow Pages when your marketing efforts consisted of a single printed advertisement within a few short pages next to every other dentist in your area code. Outbound marketing techniques were akin to training for sprints. But dentistry is more like a marathon, and these days patients demand more. The shift toward inbound marketing has placed a premium on interactive communication, unmatched customer service, transparency and delivering true value on a consistent basis. Businesses – dental offices included – must earn their customer's interest rather than purchase it. While this business model requires a greater input of time and effort, its fruit bears more loyal customers, or in your case, loyal patients. Worth your time? You bet.

Social media, combined with your unique skillset and internal marketing, builds a trusting relationship with your patients. Note the mention of your dentistry and internal resources. This book plays no part in improving your crown preps or administering anesthesia. It probably won't turn your office's Negative Nancy into Positive Patty and I can't promise that every patient who walks into your office will leave convinced that you are the one for them. Especially when considering that there are many patients who still believe a cleaning is a cleaning and a filling is a filling, no matter what dentist you go to. While we know that is not true, patients can't always assess the quality of our dentistry. But they can *always* assess their overall experience and certain objective parameters such as costs, office location, atmosphere, decor, etc. You are still responsible for the interaction while the patient is in your dental chair. Social media, on the other hand, helps keep you connected while your patient *isn't* in the chair. It keeps you relevant.

In fact, it is the most effective way to broadcast the experience of being your patient. Why? Because it tells a story. Unlike your website, which is a relatively stagnant entity, your practice's social media is a dynamic entity. I'm surprised by how many dental websites have a bio about the doctor(s) with a photo from when they graduated dental school – decades ago! They look nothing like their "profile" picture! Or think of it this way. If I'm looking for a new restaurant to try out, I'll have a few in my area to choose from. I might look at their reviews or the websites but what really seals the deal for me is if I can find photos of some of the current menu items. That way I know exactly what to expect and may even have my order ready. No surprises. By viewing your Facebook page, your patients can see snapshots around the office from yesterday or even *today*. It's almost like a journal or a photo album for your practice. It is what sets you apart – your value proposition, your *why*.

Social media is especially relevant for small and local service businesses such as a private dental office because it allows you to get personal. As I've said throughout the book, you and your staff are your practice's most unique and valuable asset. Presumably, if patients come to your office for their oral health needs, they already like you. Share photos of your staff, your family, your pets, weekend hobbies and behind-the-scenes footage at the office. People are interested in other people, and social media personifies businesses, closing the communication gap between providers and consumers.

At the end of the day, social media is simply a digital form of human interaction. The most popular content on social media exhibits the same qualities and characteristics that make other humans likeable. They are kind, witty and entertaining. They are smart, charming, empathetic. They pay you compliments and build you up. They don't criticize or complain. They are giving. They express themselves. Sometimes bold, other times thoughtful. Never fake. Always authentic.

If your dental practice has been absent from the social media table, your dinner's getting cold. The good news is that you can still join in on the fun. It's new enough to be a growing and thriving platform, but it's been around long enough that we know what works and what doesn't. Whether you are new to the scene or have enjoyed a lively online presence for years, I hope you were able to add a few social media pearls to your collection.

Based on your location, staff, office atmosphere and patient demographic you may have to alter a few variables to optimize them for your office. It is far from an exhaustive list but it's a great place to start. The particularly astute and creative readers will also expand on these concepts to various other aspects of their practice, from internal and external marketing to relating and communicating with their patients.

Pardon me if there are any outdated details on any of the platforms mentioned. Everything is up-to-date as of this writing, but social media is a rapidly evolving playground. Your practice methods, techniques and materials evolve – don't let your marketing get stagnant. Keep it fresh, try new things and have some fun!

I would like to thank you for your readership and wish you all continued growth and success. I have created a Facebook page profile (creatively) called *John Syrbu DDS*. Follow me on there so we can keep the conversation going and continue to improve our online presence together. I also look forward to your questions, feedback and comments to help guide future content. Let's keep in touch!

"Thank you."

ACKNOWLEDGEMENTS

First and foremost I would like to voice my sincere appreciation for every dentist and dental office that appears in this book. Your passion for dentistry and generosity have brought life to the text and I had a lot of fun working with you.

I would also like to extend my gratitude to the educators and mentors that I have learned so much from over the past few years. From my professors in dental school to other colleagues in the dental field. Some of you I have had the privilege of meeting in person, others I have yet to meet. It is an honor to share in the profession of dentistry with you all.

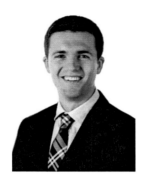

ABOUT THE AUTHOR

John Syrbu earned his B.S. in Biology from the University of Iowa and his D.D.S. from the University of Iowa College of Dentistry and Dental Clinics. John currently resides and practices in the Twin Cities area with his wife, Natalie, and their dog, Bella.

John has been illustrating dental cartoons since his first year of dental school and incorporates them into a Facebook page he created called *Dental Art & Humor*. A collection of his comics can be found in a book with the same title. Other works by John include *The Complete Pre-Dental Guide to Modern Dentistry* and *Tommy the Tooth: Tommy's New Friend*. John also enjoys speaking engagements with a variety of audiences. He can be reached at john.syrbu@gmail.com or private message to his Facebook page.

Made in United States
North Haven, CT
21 April 2022

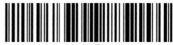

18436576R00066